1

Copyright Page

Blossom's FearLess Journal: A Path Toward Courage
Copyright © 2020 by
Tamara Hall Fuchs

Blossom's FearLess Journal
A Path toward Courage

An Integrative Health Coach in a Book

By Tamara Hall Fuchs

Photography:
Thomas and Tamara Hall Fuchs

Editor:
George Boesger

Graphic Design:
Thomas B. Fuchs & Summer Derrickson

Illustrator:
Summer's Art Studio
1summernightmedia.com

Group and Classroom Discounts Available
BlossomsFearLess@gmail.com

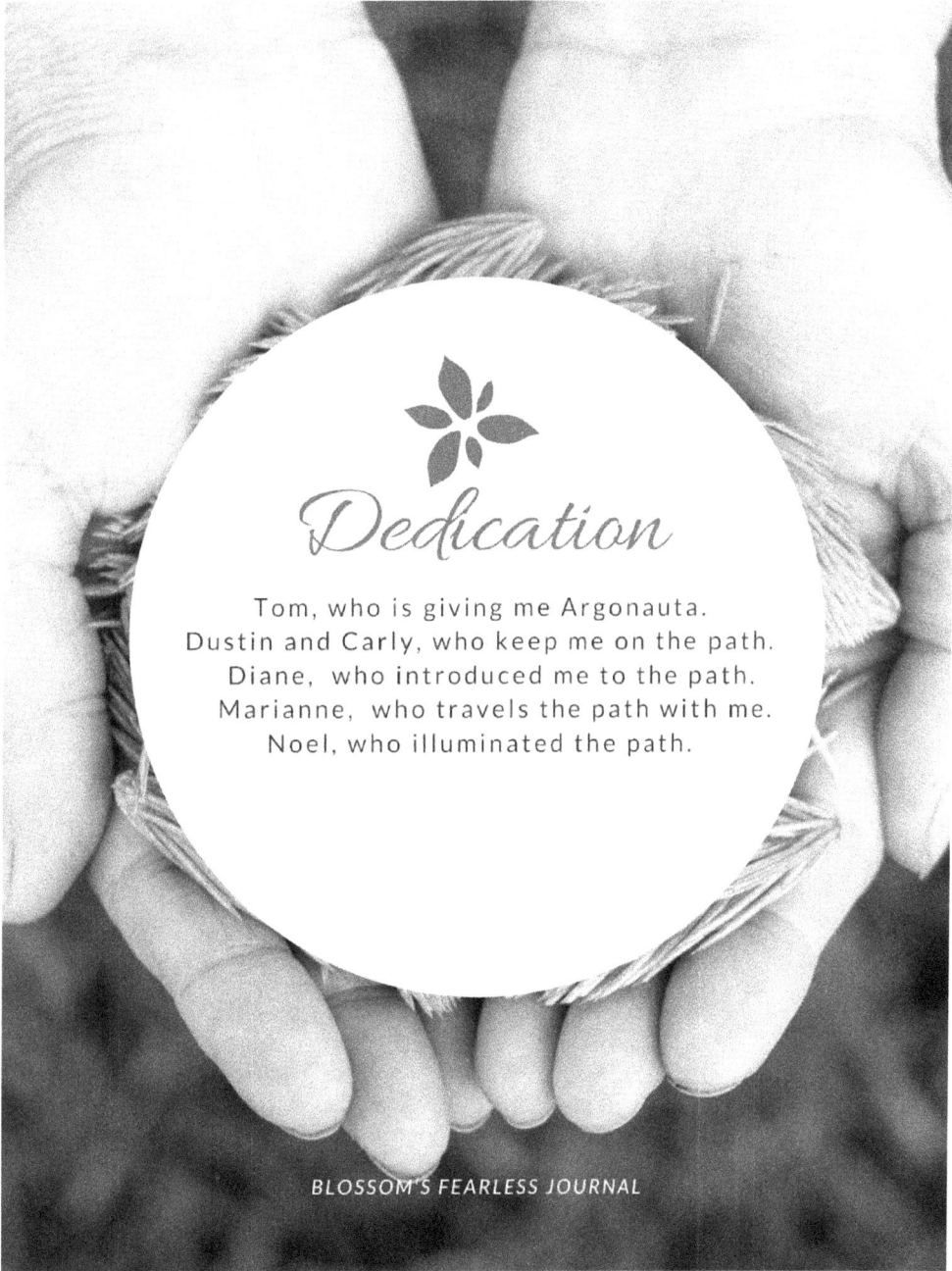

Dedication

Tom, who is giving me Argonauta.
Dustin and Carly, who keep me on the path.
Diane, who introduced me to the path.
Marianne, who travels the path with me.
Noel, who illuminated the path.

BLOSSOM'S FEARLESS JOURNAL

In Gratitude

Renee Grandi, Racheal Karlin
Stephen Kliewer, Noel Busby , TaiMarie Jaques, Patricia Zennie
Barbara Tyler, Kelly Boeve, Elizabeth Powers
John Suto, Billy Suto. Darold Bigger,
Max Hammonds, Carolyn Hammonds, Terri Hall Haskins
James E Harri,   Kelly Casey, Colleen Whalen,
Kate Forester, Amy Zahn, Kate Barrett, Andrea Haney
Lisa Dawson, Laura Dees, Kana Oliver, Shirley Holmes
Heather Hall Tourville, Joy Estock

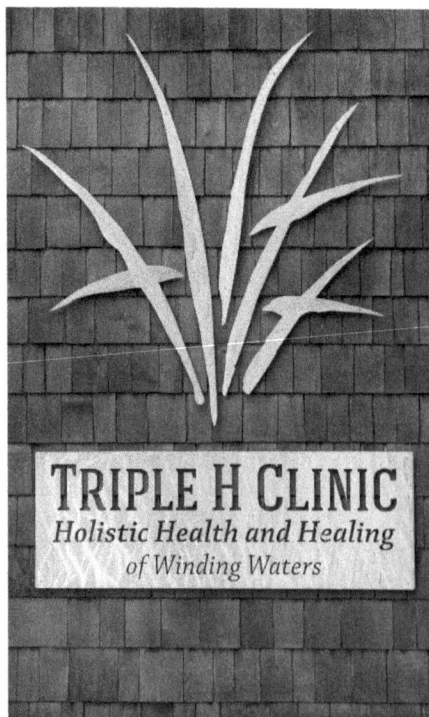

TRIPLE H CLINIC
Holistic Health and Healing
of Winding Waters

Gratitude to Wallowa County

I am very grateful for all the leaders, organizations, and private citizens that have supported us and kept us safe during this Covid-19 Global Crisis. So many have stepped up to the plate, sacrificed, and made the difficult decisions necessary to safeguard our health and welfare. Small rural communities have limited resources to ensure the health of their residents, so it's critical that these resources coordinate and cooperates in dire times of need. We have seen medical providers, business owners, and law enforcement join forces to combat the spread of the virus and rise to the occasion, often at their own risk and expense. I am proud to call
Wallowa County home.

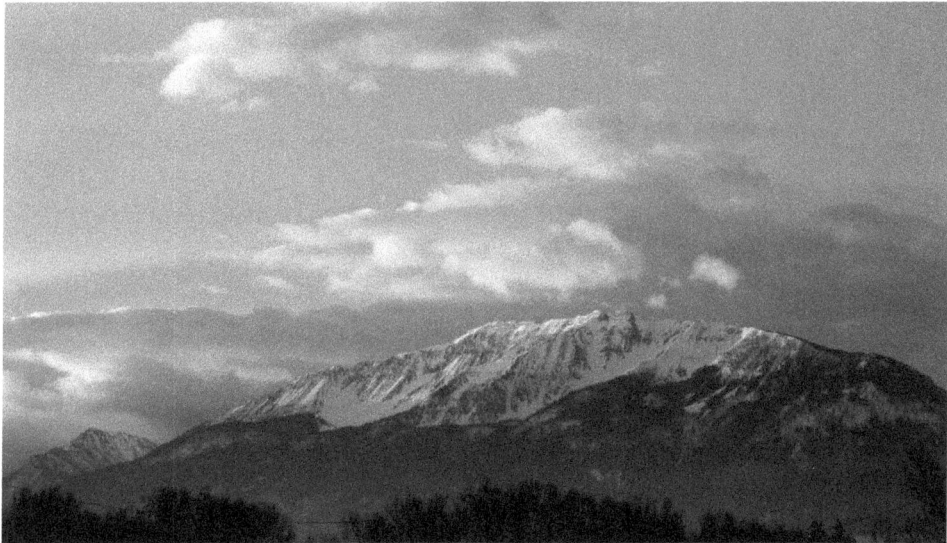

Blossom's FearLess Journal

A Journey toward Courage

Forward: Dr. Stephen Kliewer

My Path Toward Courage

How To Use This Book

Healing Habits

Your Path Toward Courage

Afterward: Noel Busby

"One of the new things people began to find out in the last century was that thoughts—just mere thoughts—are as powerful as electric batteries—as good for one as sunlight is, or as bad for one as poison. To let a sad thought or a bad one get into your mind is as dangerous as letting a scarlet fever germ get into your body. If you let it stay there after it has got in you may never get over it as long as you live... surprising things can happen to anyone who, when a disagreeable or discouraged thought comes into his mind, just has the sense to remember in time and push it out by putting in an agreeable determinedly courageous one. Two things cannot be in one place."

"Where you tend a rose, my lad, A thistle cannot grow."

~ Frances Hodgson Burnett, 1911, The Secret Garden

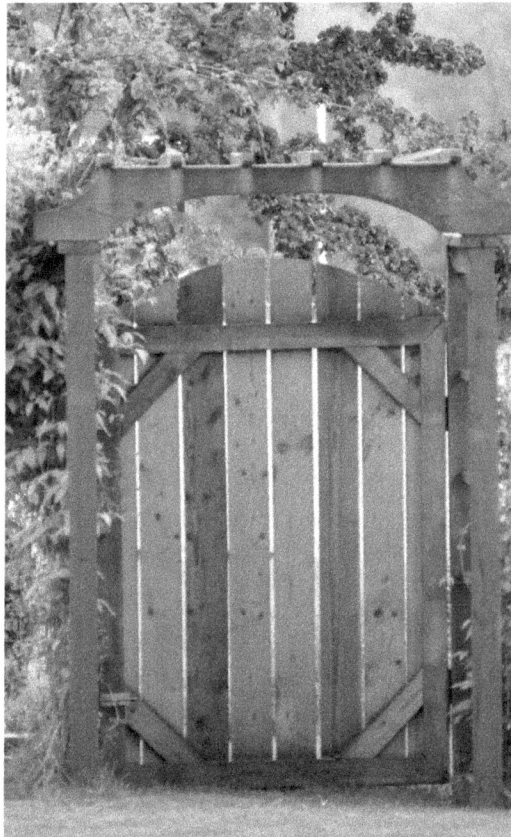

Forward

There is no question about it. Life can be difficult. It seems at times as if no matter how hard we work, how many tools we amass, there is always "something" that comes along to create pain. That pain can take many forms.

Sometimes it is physical. At other times it is mental, emotional, or spiritual. Sometimes that pain turns to suffering. Pain is unavoidable. Relationships end, bodies get ill, tragedies happen. We all experience pain at one time or another, but suffering is optional. Suffering is the way we respond to our pain, doubling if not tripling the effects of the pain itself. Suffering is when our physical ailment causes us to start thinking less of ourselves as human beings, when failure becomes not simply the result of choices that we make, but proof that positive we are a failure.

Sometimes, when we get caught up in suffering, we get stuck. We fall into "patterned responses." Thoughts come into our heads unbidden and automatic. Feelings too. We don't choose these responses; they just come somewhat automatically. Out of those patterned inner responses come patterned external responses. We behave in predictable and often problematic ways. Feeling insecure, we isolate. Feeling sad, we eat. Feeling unworthy, we torment ourselves.

However, we have an amazing tool available to us: awareness. When we learn to step away from our "bully brains" and notice what we are thinking and feeling and how we are responding, we once again claim personal power. We can find that flexibility that allows us to get unstuck and move down the path toward growth and the full expression of our True Selves.Tamara Hall Fuchs is a person who has gone to health hell and back. She has experienced debilitating health issues, compounded by uncertainty and confusion. She has struggled with the impact of a difficult childhood and toxic influences on her life. Through it all, however, she has, to use her own words, "blossomed."

She has moved from a place of being overwhelmed and frozen by her issues into a place where she can now reach out with wisdom and compassion to others who are in their own "stuck places." She has worked hard to understand herself, educate herself, and heal herself. Following a career as a health teacher and neurodiversity specialist, she has returned to school and become internationally certified as an integrative health coach. She has put her learning into practice, using food, mindfulness, and other natural tools to heal. She has worked collaboratively with other local healers, physicians, therapists, and others to develop an approach that can lead to lifestyle change and healing.

I have worked with Tamara Hall Fuchs for many years and have seen her at many different stages in this journey. I was present in her life when some of her health and emotional issues first flared up and watched as she struggled with both diagnoses and misdiagnoses. I also watched as she was impacted physically, mentally, and spiritually and pushed to the edge of despair. In the aftermath of her struggle to reclaim her wellness, I witnessed her gathering people around her, collecting wisdom, learning tools, and fighting her way back to the place where she could be a person who contributes to her community.

One of the most wonderful things about Tamara Hall Fuchs is her deep desire to help other people. This is why she was a teacher, why she worked with children struggling with mental health issues, why she chose to become a health coach, and why she serves the community in many different ways.

The transformation in Tamara's life has been remarkable. I remember seeing her as she emerged from the deepest and darkest moments and moved toward health and being stunned by the difference in how her body looked. Her previous patently unhealthy pallor now glowed with healthfulness. I was moved, too, by the difference in her voice, a voice that had been silenced and then distorted, but now was back. Her eyes, once fearful and despair, are now full of life.

I know that if she can use this process to reclaim herself, others can too. I hope you will take the time to use this book carefully. Be patient with yourself and with the process. Growth is difficult, change is scary, and blossoming takes time, but it is all possible with awareness, flexibility, and the power that is within you!

Stephen Kliewer, M.Div. D.Min. M.S. Mental Health Counseling 7/7/2020 Stephen Kliewer has degrees in English Literature, Philosophy, Theology, and Psychology Dr. Stephen Kliewer's experiences are varied. He has been as a pastor, has worked as an EMT and disaster relief worker, has been on the faculty at a medical school (Oregon Health and Science University), and, for the past 18 years, has been a mental health professional. For 13 years, he was the director of a community mental health program and has served as a therapist as a licensed professional counselor. Dr. Kliewer has authored three books, one on diversity, one on spirituality and health, and a soon-to-be-published work on journaling the spiritual, psychological, and ethical issues of our current world. His relationship with the author is both personal and professional and goes back over a decade.

My Path toward Courage

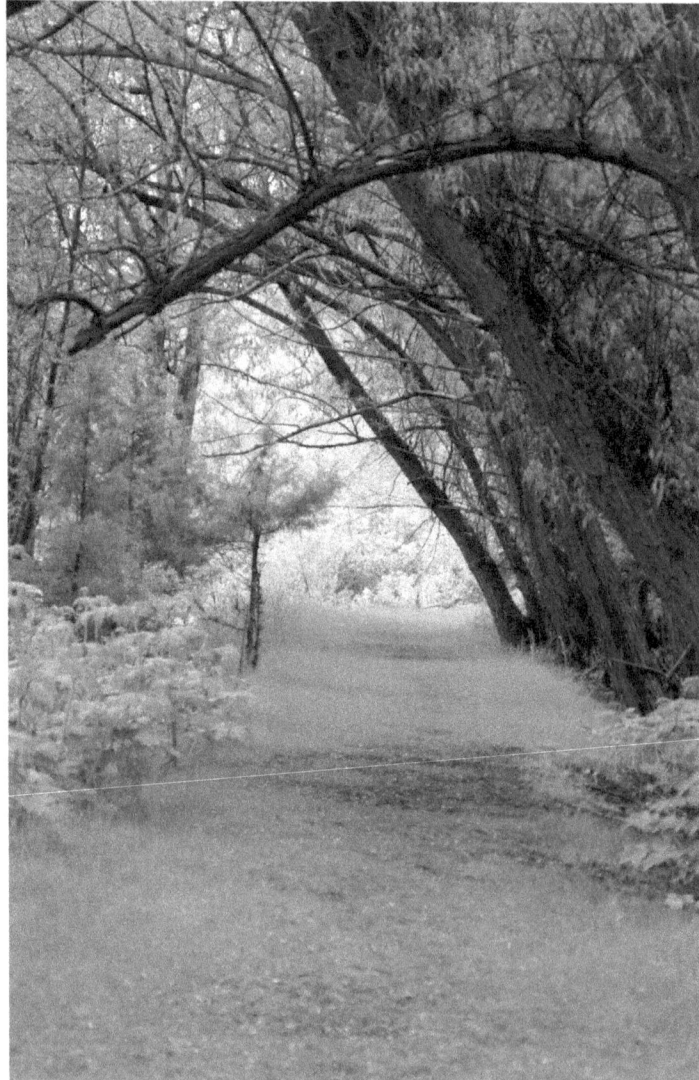

Being truly human, transforming the profane into the sacred, is the ultimate alchemy.

~A. Schultz

This is my story of how, at first, I was gripped by a compelling fear of life and how my life transformed into what it is today. It's a challenging story to tell and read, one that has taken my entire life to tell. My path has led me through some dark places, but in the end, that same path has brought me to a place of light-filled courageous fearlessness. I would like to tell you how fear debilitated me, provide examples of those fears, explain how my life has been transformed through gratitude and grace, and offer suggestions on how, through gratitude, you might transform your own life to one of grace-filled peace and joy.

My story begins with a colossal challenge related to a plethora of medical conditions that at times seemed totally out of control. It seemed that every other week, I was pronounced with a new and dire medical diagnosis. With each pronouncement, fear crept into my psyche like a brain-eating scavenger. My life no longer belonged to me. It belonged to a gripping and unrelenting fear. These out-of-control medical challenges caused physical distortions of my physical being, and one challenge led to another in what became an unending stream of toxic waste flooding my life. For example, after a heart attack in 2012, I also had a stroke in 2014. This was followed by cauda equina and a series of back surgeries caused by a previous auto accident. The surgeries necessitated two nursing home stays and multiple hospitalizations. In the middle of all of this medical mayhem, I also was diagnosed with multiple autoimmune disorders, pre-diabetes and insulin resistance, non-alcoholic fatty liver disease, sleep apnea, migraine headaches, adrenal fatigue, severe arthritis, and degenerative disc disease. My life at that point felt like a never-ending, ever-intensifying nightmare. This culminated in 2016, when the doctor delivered the worst possible news: the diagnosis of colon cancer. My countless medical maladies were spinning out of control, and something had to be done to rescue not only my physical well-being but my psychic plunge into the depths of despair.

The series of medical conditions had taken their toll on the more exterior aspects of my personal life as well. I had been a single mother for years, but my physical obstacles caused my children to live with their father. I also had to give up my professional career. Ironically, I had been a health teacher in various capacities for years. I felt that I knew how to be healthy, but I was unable to lose weight even though I had been following the food pyramid and the science available at the time, even with the aid of nutritionists and dieticians. My family's negative health history was also a clanging bell demanding attention, but my efforts to manage my perplexing medical conditions failed.

In the meantime, I had reconnected with my high school and college sweetheart, so I wanted to do more than merely exist; I wanted to THRIVE. It seemed that I needed to exercise more patience for that to manifest, however, though hope was on the horizon. As I sat in my doctor's office in February of 2017, I did not realize my life was going to transform into something that I could not have even imagined. My doctor suggested yet another diet. This one was to address inflammation and eliminate various foods to support a better understanding of my food sensitivities and allergies. Cutting out sugar, grains, legumes, dairy, and alcohol seemed absurd at the time, but it has healed my body and taken me back to my adolescent body size. This new diet regime revolutionized my entire life. In addition to losing significant weight, the diet corrected the fatty liver disease, reversed pre-diabetes, and relieved sleep apnea. It turned out that finding the answers to how food affects our bodies was the key. Much of what was happening with my reactivity to foods was based on extreme sensitivities to chemicals and preservatives. Now that I exclusively eat organically grown food, virtually all of that reactivity has been reversed.

I thought my health issues were addressed, so I was ready for a more complete transformation. However, I experienced a setback with a new cancer diagnosis that at first was devastating to the point that I began end-of-life legal proceedings. Oregon permits death with dignity, so the process itself was not difficult to accomplish. The grueling reality facing me became my turning point. After researching and earnestly seeking wholeness, I latched onto what became my eventual answer. All of this time, fear is what prompted me to act: fear of extreme illness, injury, dire pain, and eventual death. I was terrified, and most of my actions were the result of that terror. The paradigm shifted when I courageously decided to find ways to be grateful for all that I had undergone. It probably sounds moonstruck to suggest gratitude in light of the extreme life-threatening illnesses mentioned here, but in many ways, those challenges brought me to the brink of no other alternative. Medical science had done its level best to diagnose and address my complex of maladies, but it fell short of fully rectifying my condition. My healthfulness had to begin and end from within, not from without. I decided to excavate my interior, discover the woman I was meant to be, to grab ahold of every possible thing to be grateful for, and get on with life. I discovered a fundamental linkage between gratitude and grace, which has come to mean something far more complex than its typical understanding.

The universe seems to love to give unexpected and undeserved presents that normally manifest as mental paradigm shifts. This generosity is what I refer to as grace. Curiously enough, gratitude is the very thing that activates grace, and once grace is realized, it in turn activates gratitude. In essence, they co-exist as cosmic dyads. When I came upon this realization, when I discovered the connection between living a life of gratitude based on grace, my whole life began to transform into one of ease, filling entire days with peace and joy. Please know that I still have my challenges. Many of the physical maladies mentioned above still afflict me. Rather than fueling my reactivity to those obstacles with fear, however, I greet them with gratitude, which diffuses and disarms their power over me. At the end of this book, you will find a list of the books, media presentations, and materials that got me through the last year.

I have walked this long path towards courage over the last 6 years. I have learned so much and my life has been transformed. During the month of February 2020, I struck out on a note of courage that has resulted in the book that you are now reading after enrolling in my last class at the Institute of Integrative Nutrition, called "Launch Your Dream Book." I had always dreamed of writing a book and had found such comfort, healing, and transformation in my journaling over the last several years. I decided to share what I had learned with others who may be facing body, mind, or soul challenges of their own.

It is my wish for you that you too can find a way to dislodge fear from your life, to courageously discover the linkage between gratitude and grace. Realistically, life may never be completely without fear. Fear is a motivator, as my life attests to. It can serve as a signal to pay attention, to find new ways of living, and to discover new perspectives on how to activate grace in our lives. The single takeaway from this message is this: A life filled with gratitude leads to a life full of peace and joy, which are the gifts that the universe provides in response to our gratitude. I encourage you to take a risk and give it a try.

How to Use This Journal

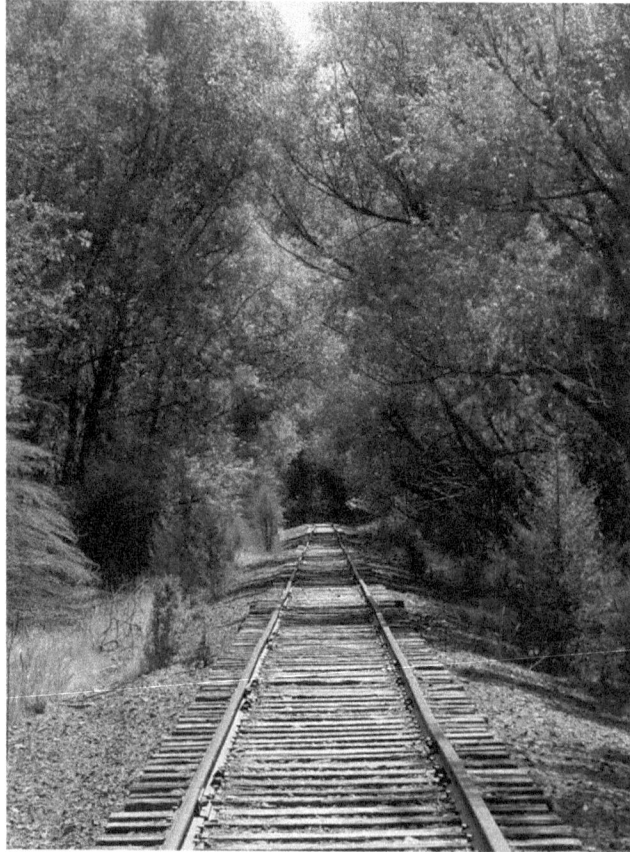

"Into a dancer, you have grown
From a see somebody else has thrown.
Go ahead and throw some seeds of your own,
And somewhere between the time you arrive
And the time you go may lie the reason you were alive.
~ Jackson Browne

Imagine you are standing in front of a newly prepared garden space. You do not know what the soil will produce. You may not be sure of where the sun shines and where the shady spots are. This is a fresh new season, and you have high hopes for a luscious and abundant crop. Your *FearLess* journal is the rich, fertile soil ready for tilling that cultivates the discovery of True Self.

Blossom's FearLess Journal is an experiential and therapeutic approach to finding balance, living with curiosity, and living your best life with courage. An integrative health coach in a book, this journal takes a bio-individual approach to whole-body health. You will be exploring and addressing physical, social, emotional, intellectual, and spiritual health. This book is organized in a way that is consistent with brain science and building change through habit tracking and daily prompts. It will lead you down a path toward inner wisdom that exists within you now but may feel very hard to find. You will discover that you have everything you need within to let your most Authentic Self shine through.

As you peer through the plants in the garden seeking ripe fruits, you will go through a carefully designed program to clarify your values and intentions. This journal will lead you to understand the motivational aspect of clearly defining your life's purpose and how to achieve it one day at a time.

As you work through the prompts and worksheets and integrate the practices offered in this journal, you will cultivate a deeper understanding of who you are. Understanding who you are and what you want out of this life will point in the direction of becoming the best YOU.

As you go down this path, you will notice yourself asking many introspective questions and be given the tools to properly address them. You will learn the source of rage or fear, joy, or niggling uncomfortable feelings. You may see things differently with time, space, and maturity, thereby giving you fresh eyes and a new perspective.

Throughout the journal, you will find the following key organizing markers to help track your progress.

● **Date:** This is to help you track your progress throughout. It is beneficial to have a written record of transformation and growth. Keeping track of your progress can become a source of wonder at the subtle nature of change.

● **Today's Intention:** Setting an intention each day reminds you of your ultimate purpose and focuses on what is important. Throughout the day you can self-evaluate by asking, "Does this move me towards my intention for my day?"

● **Healing Habit Tracker:** Sleep, plenty of water, good oral hygiene, movement, meditation, and breathing exercises are all small tools that have a major impact on overall health and wellness. Like watering a garden to support lush, rich growth, you also must attend to small daily habits to attain and maintain your highest level of physical, emotional, and intellectual health. This box is positioned in the lower outside corner of your journal pages, so if you notice a health concern, you can flip back and see if there are small habits that you have missed consistently.

- **Daily Prompt:** Each day has a prompt to stimulate a systematic approach towards discovering your True Self. These prompts are thematically based on the focus of each month but are also designed to lead you to dig deeper than you would alone. Brain science teaches us about the plasticity of the brain and how introspection is the most efficient way to get to the answers that can change our lives.

- **My Mantra:** Here is where you can create a mantra that is an act of choosing love each day. It can be something that you feel will support you through the day, either in your words or something that inspires you. This positive affirmation is a powerful way to let go of fear and start your day with a positive mindset.

- **Gratitude:** I believe that gratitude manifests grace. Grace allows for a free-flowing life, and a grateful disposition invites grace. We have all had days where it seems impossible to unlock a door, and others where things just seem to fall into place. This is the grace we are aiming for: flowing through life freely and with little effort.

- **Concerns, Opportunities, Outcome**: This feature is a worry tracker. Here, you can write out your fears and possible solutions. You can also note your fears or worries about possible outcomes. The journal daily page also provides a visual reminder that you are a problem-solver and you can successfully move through past trauma or fear.

- **Quote or Recommendation:** A quote will prompt your meditation practice or sharpen your focus as you walk through your day. These prompts are short bits of wisdom to help you frame questions and interpret their answers. Recommendations take the shape of book titles, online suggestions, or other motivational tools.

- **Life Skill Worksheets:** The skills outlined here are what we all need to support healthy interpersonal relationships, personal quests for the right answers within ourselves, and transformational personal growth in exploring our life's purpose. These practical skills are ones we use often in life, but schools' emphasis on standardized testing rather than life-skill development has missed the mark on whole-person development. These worksheets fill the gap by addressing a more holistically transformed version of our True Selves.

- **Book Recommendations:** You will find a listing at the back of the book of the books that I have used for my own personal transformation. Some are common books that I've used over the last 3 years. Others are favorites from a lifetime of being an avid reader. Each book speaks to the theme of each chapter and may be a self-help book or a selection from children's literature that you can share with a child or grandchild to pass on enlightenment and important life lessons to a younger set of friends.

- **Self-Care Challenge:** I have included a tracking form that you can fill in with a month of self-care to support further personal growth and to feed your choice for self-compassion. Many of us lead very busy lives and we seem to put ourselves at the bottom of the list. Self-Compassion is the tool for you to use to live your best life and find your True Self.

Healing Habits

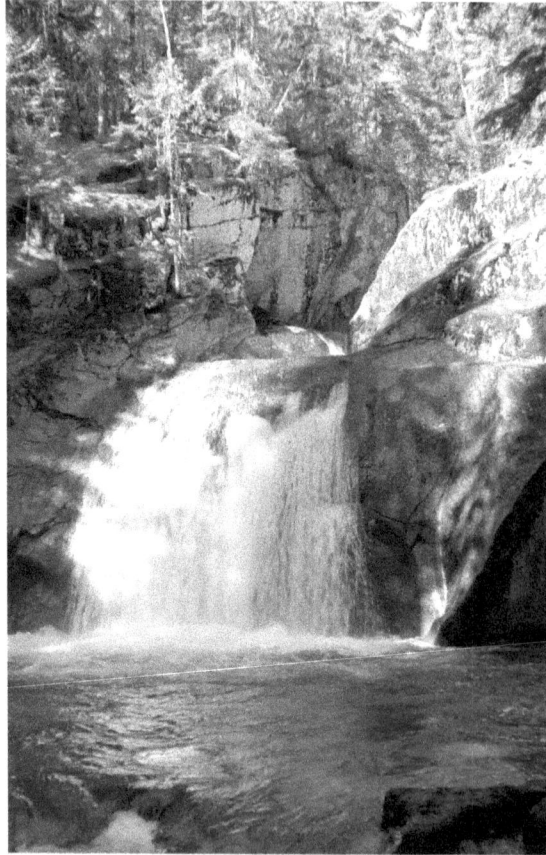

Without a doubt, healthful routines improve our quality of life. In fact, they all but ensure a vibrant life. Healing habits only take root and sprout when performed ritualistically and consistently. It may seem tedious at first, but routines that heal our bodies guarantee the outcome of the best version of yourself. They affect both how we feel as well as our appearance. They can also overhaul our interactions with others and our view of life.

I rehearse my gardening within by performing it without. Here in Oregon, gardening season is especially short and intense. Every Spring, I plan my every move in my backyard garden. I plan the planting and cultivating of every plant, making sure that each of them gets the sunlight and water they need. After the initial design is set out for the garden and its beds are established, the maintenance of the growing season is relaxed. Over the course of the summer growing season, I even plan meals according to what the garden produces that week. Every morning at the break of dawn, I visit my garden, scoping every new growth, watering, and pruning to maximize growth. I have found that maintaining a regular watering schedule is the biggest factor in whether the garden will thrive. Our health is remarkably similar, which is one reason it's so easy to neglect. Suddenly, you may find yourself chronically ill or living a life dominated by fear.

I have meditated on the inner and outer healthy habits that yield growth in my life. I would like to share them with you here:

Sleep - Sleep is essential for living a healthy life. If you've ever had periods of interrupted sleep you know and understand the impact of lack of sleep, whether it be from your job, a new baby, a sick child, or a deadline for work that keeps you up. Maintaining a good sleep schedule and making sleep a priority goes far in supporting you on your path towards a better life. Tracking your sleep quality and quantity is helpful in deciphering issues that come up in our daily lives.

Clean Eating - After sleep, food is, by far, the most impactful in healthy living. However, there are no simple rules for this; each individual needs to define "clean eating" for her or himself. Being aware of the body's reaction to food is the key and tracking these reactions through journaling is one way to discover "clean eating" for yourself. My doctors and I have collaborated on classes in our community to encourage the use of science to heal our bodies with an anti-inflammatory, elimination diet. For me, clean eating means no processed foods, less than 6 teaspoons of sugar in my daily diet and eating organic foods. We are each different. I use the term bio-individual often to mean that your body is unique and works differently than other bodies.

Move Your Body - Once we have a healthy sleep routine in place and have incorporated "clean eating" in our diet, physical activity is next in line for overall health. Moving our bodies is a healthy way to release pent up negative energy. Of course, it also keeps our bodies in peak performance mode, which also contributes to an engaged life. If you have given up caffeine and still feel an inner buzz that simply will not go away try jumping on your bike or into a lake, or anything that ignites your breath. Personally, I use yoga daily to check in with my body and move, gain strength, and explore my physical health. I ride my bike, aiming for a 5-minute mile to release pent up energy, which, in turn, helps to burn calories and fosters a good night's sleep.

Water - Our bodies are bombarded by noise, dirt, and toxins on a daily if not momentary level. We are essentially surrounded by the things that make us sick, in some cases, morbidly so. Having a healthy sleeping, resting, and exercise regime in place does a lot to ward off this barrage of badness, but one more thing is essential: water. Clean, pure, unadulterated water. In fact, water is our first line of defense when it comes to supporting our livers and immune systems. It aids in clearing out what our bodies do not need and cannot use to support vibrant health. Drinking sufficient water goes far in supporting a clean system that can operate at its best.

Breathing Exercises - Meditation gurus often tell us to enter the room of meditation through our senses. What do we hear or smell? How does the cushion that you are sitting on feel? As we allow our senses to register the reality surrounding us, it is deep, regular breathing that brings inner stillness. It also raises a sense of inner balance and peace to a completely different level. The quiet time you spend with your yoga instructor or by following a reputable program will add clarity and composure to your mental state, allowing you to process information and calm your anxiety. This whole thing takes practice, however. It took me nearly a year to integrate a breathing focus into my yoga practice on a consistent basis. It took another year for me to realize how much better my practice became when my breathing and movement were synced. I reaped the full benefits of a daily yoga practice which includes, for me, clarity of thought and inner peace. At the back of this book, I have recommended a Wim Hof video in the recommendations to help you explore this possibility if it seems of interest.

Oral Health - This is one of the most overlooked and underrated aspects of overall health. Healthy oral habits not only contribute to one's overall wellness; they can also keep us from unnecessary and expensive visits to the dentist! Probably the quickest way to deteriorate one's oral health is by night-time grinding of teeth, which is a symptom of pent up anxiety. The breathing exercise mentioned above can do a lot to assuage teeth grinding, but a good mouthguard will protect one's teeth during particularly stressful times. When fear is deep, we can grind out teeth so hard during sleep that we crack or break our teeth. Maintaining excellent oral hygiene during times of fear-driven physical manifestations is a simple way to keep your teeth from adding to crisis.

Visualization - Our internal eye is a powerful tool to help us create a peaceful and calm reality. I use visualization daily in a focused way for a set amount of time to change my brain pathways for a more positive mindset and healing. On days when I have a task that I am uncomfortable with but must perform, I often rehearse difficult interactions with others through visualization ahead of time. For instance, I had an exceedingly difficult conversation earlier this year and I practiced it in writing. Afterward, I imagined having that conversation, using different approaches to achieve the greatest possibility of understanding. This allowed me to work through my spoken stumbles toward a respectful yet assertive delivery. Through visualization, I can anticipate, explore, and practice various ways to meet my intention with kindness and grace. The other use of visualization comes from Anne Hopper of Dynamic Neural Retraining Systems and provides a retraining of brainwave patterns to break free of default fear-based responses. Many of us have fear-based emotional response pathways deep in our brains. Brain retraining can support changing those pathways to break the patterns of fear we have learned throughout our lives.

Emotional Response Awareness - How we automatically respond to what happens in our day is a huge indicator of our brains work. If we automatically blame, judge, and rage toward others, we may be using old brain pathways that no longer serve us. Changing our automatic responses takes time. There are ways to focus on developing more positive emotional response systems. By focusing our awareness of fear in our lives, we can choose a loving response instead by seeing things through a positive lens. If we are strolling through our neighborhood after dinner do, we see the brokenness around us or do we see beauty? Awareness of your "go-to" responses is the first step in changing from a negative, fear-based mindset to a positive or love-based one. Choose love and let go of fear.

Solitude - To truly be in touch with our True Self, we must take quiet time alone to explore what the right answers truly are for us. Developmentally, most of us go through a phase early in life of asking everyone else opinions about what we should or should not do. We know we have positive emotional maturity when we realize that we are really the only one that knows what is right for us. Ironically, taking time to be alone during the day can garner better sleep at night. I have found if I don't take quiet time each day, I wake up throughout the night with my subconscious trying to get my attention and give me the answers I've not taken the quiet time to listen for during the day.

Lymph Drainage - Our bodies in the Twenty First Century are overwrought with tension and toxins. Clamor and poisons abound. Our lymph system is our body's way of collecting toxins, but it does not have a pumping system of its own. To expel toxins from our lymph system, we must move our bodies through physical activity such as yoga and get regular massages. I have adopted a simple morning routine of dry body brushing before I get in the shower. I then wash my hair and body while focusing on the areas where lymph collects such as either side of my throat, my armpits, and backs of my knees. Afterward, I put on body lotion and make sure to stroke towards my middle to support excellent lymph drainage. Massaging and draining my lymph system supports my body in daily detoxing.

Awareness - It is essential that we remain fully aware in body, mind, and spirit as well as all areas of life. Many of us blindly trust medical professionals who may or may not have our best interest in mind. It is vital to seek answers to the CAUSE of your health challenges and treat them at that level, rather than throwing pharmaceuticals at them. If you do use pharmaceuticals, please verify their use at DRUGS.COM to check for full information and correct indications of the drug. After all, we must live with our bodies, so it is up to us to take responsibility for our health and wellness by implementing healthy habits each day.

my intentions

	Where I am	Where I want to be.	Action Plan

Physical

Emotional

Social

Intellectual

Spiritual

Professional

my intentions

	Where I am	Where I want to be.	Action Plan
Physical			
Emotional			
Social			
Intellectual			
Spiritual			
Professional			

Choose Love
Let Go of Fear

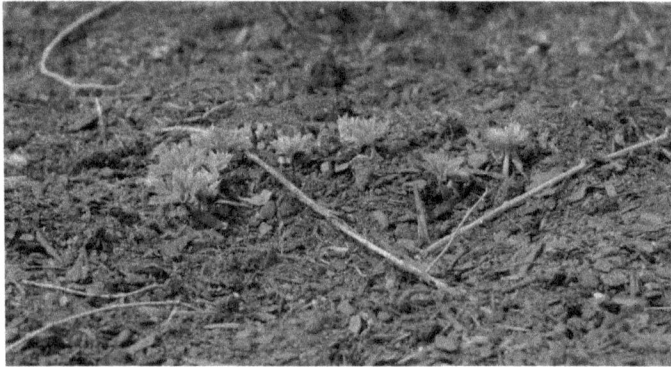

"Fearlessness may be a gift but perhaps the more precious thing is the courage acquired through endeavor, courage that comes from cultivating the habit of refusing to let fear dictate one's actions, courage that could be described as 'grace under pressure'- grace which is renewed repeatedly in the face of harsh, unremitting pressure."

~ Aung San Suu Kyi

"The doctor's question rang throughout my head."

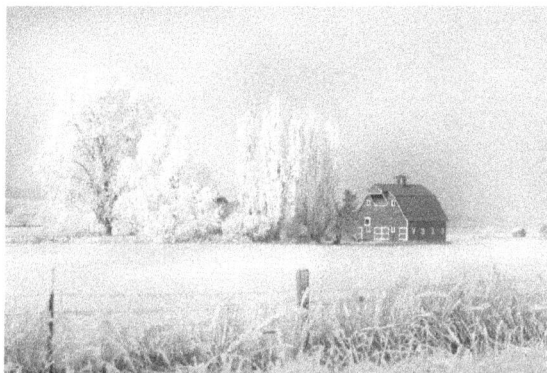

My life has been one enormous topsy turvy ride, starting with a thwarted childhood and young adulthood, stemming into one medically-related midlife crisis after another, finally ending on a note of deeply yearned for peace and joy. It's been quite a ride, one that I would never wish on anyone. But getting to this point requires a bit of explanation. In the end, I hope that my journey will encourage you to strike out and secure your own sense of True Self.

That morning, the doctor's question resounded throughout my head. "What if nothing's wrong with you?" Fear flooded my entire being and ice ran in my veins. No, I want a known and sure diagnosis. I did not want to go back to the unknown. The thought that I'd been misdiagnosed was overwhelming. The question enraged me. I thought we were through this part. I didn't even want to consider ANY OTHER OPTION. My doctor knew what I did not. Many of my "neuroendocrine tumor" (NET) symptoms were physical manifestations of fear. Sleepless nights, tears constantly running down my face, digestive upset and years of constant diarrhea, odd lightning-strike headaches, confused thinking, panic attacks, "cotton brain," forgetting words, speaking in "stroke voice," all of these were signs I have come to recognize as fear.

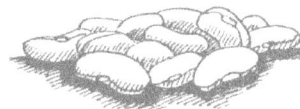

For those nights when sleep eludes you, keep a small tablet by the bed to write down what you'll need to remember the next day - then let it go and return to sleep.

Chronic illness can be a wicked stepmother, one that demands attention at every waking moment. However, we are not our illness and health challenges. That is just one part of us. The more we maintain our sense of Self, despite our diagnosis, the quicker we will heal. And if we don't heal completely or immediately, we will adjust our lives to make them work for us. The choice is ours to make. Either we can choose love and a positive mindset, explore solutions, or, we can allow our illness to identify as ourselves, causing us to live in fear, rather than love.

If your life has become unmanageable by chronic illness, you have some decisions to make about how to coexist with your maladies. With research and inner exploration, you will know what is right for you and how much time you want to dedicate to your recovery. Essentially the choice is yours to make. Either we live an incapacitated life based in fear, or we live an engaged life based in love. It's that simple, yet that profound. I choose to engage in love. I invite you to do the same.

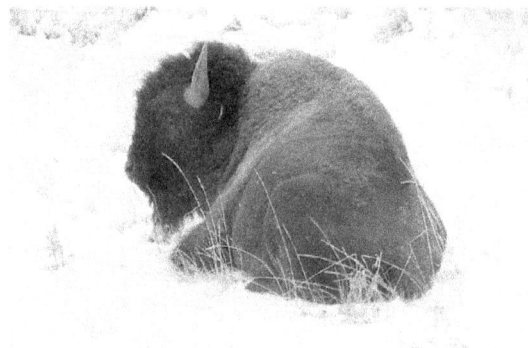

33

Date: Today's Intention:

As an expression of love, who am I? How
can I express love today?

Gratitude: Celebrations/Concerns:

                                         Opportunities:

"The most exhausting thing in life, I have discovered, is
being insincere."
        - Anne Morrow Lindbergh, Gift from the Sea

Healing Habits: My Mantra:

    Water   Movement
    Meditation   Sleep
    Clean Eating   Visualize
    Oral Health   Quiet Alone

Today's Intention: Date:

How can i be of support love towards another today?

Celebrations/Concerns: Gratitude:

Opportunities:

"Don't be afraid of death be afraid of an unlived life
You don't have to live forever, you just have to live."
- Natalie Babbitt

My Mantra: Healing Habits:
                                          Water   Movement
                                          Meditation   Sleep
                                          Clean Eating   Visualize
                                          Oral Health   Quiet Alone

Date:

Today's Intention:

How will love manifest in my life today?

Gratitude:

Celebrations/Concerns:

Opportunities:

"Our deepest fear is not that we are
inadequate. Our deepest fear is that we are
powerful beyond measure. It is our light, not
our darkness, that most frightens us."
                                    - Marianne Williamson

Healing Habits:

My Mantra:

   Water   Movement
   Meditation   Sleep
   Clean Eating   Visualize
   Oral Health   Quiet Alone

Today's Intention: Date:

With whom do i feel most able to let my light shine? What
is love?

Celebrations/Concerns: Gratitude:

Opportunities

"Learn to let go. That is the key to happiness"
                                              ~ The Buddha

My Mantra: Healing Habits:
                                                 Water   Movement
                                                 Meditation   Sleep
                                                 Clean Eating   Visualize
                                                 Oral Health   Quiet Alone

Date: Today's Intention:

How will love manifest in my life today?

Gratitude: Celebrations/Concerns:

Opportunities:

"Journaling is a cornerstone habit. When practiced daily, journaling has the ability to transform other parts of your life powerfully."

~ Charles Durhigg

Healing Habits: My Mantra:

Water   Movement
Meditation   Sleep
Clean Eating   Visualize
Oral Health   Quiet Alone

Today's Intention: Date:

Consider fear to be a cloud, something that is diaphanous
and floats by, not a part of us, but there sometimes. How
does this change my perception of fear? If I feel fear,
can I use it as a signal to problem-solve with a positive
mindset?

Celebrations/Concerns: Gratitude:

Opportunities:

"You don't have to be who you first were."
" Jen Hatmaker

My Mantra: Healing Habits:
                                                  Water   Movement
                                                  Meditation   Sleep
                                                  Clean Eating   Visualize
                                                  Oral Health   Quiet Alone

Date:

How does my body signal that I am experiencing fear?

Gratitude:

Celebrations/Concerns:

Opportunities:

"Expect trouble as an inevitable part of life, and when it comes, hold your head high, look it squarely in the eye and say, 'I will be bigger than you. You cannot defeat me.'"

-Anne Landers

Healing Habits:

Water   Movement
Meditation   Sleep
Clean Eating Visualize
Oral Health Quiet Alone

My Mantra:

Today's Intention: Date:

How do I make myself feel safe?

Celebrations/Concerns: Gratitude:

Opportunities:

"An affirmation is a strong positive statement that
something is already so."

~ Shakti Gawain

My Mantra: Healing Habits:

.   Water   Movement
                                               Meditation   Sleep
                                               Clean Eating   Visualize
                                               Oral Health   Quiet Alone

Date: Today's Intention:

How can I best thrive today?

Gratitude: Celebrations/Concerns:

                                       Opportunities:

"Only love can be divided endlessly and still not
diminish."
              — Anne Morrow Lindbergh

Healing Habits: My Mantra:

   Water   Movement
   Meditation   Sleep
   Clean Eating Visualize
   Oral Health Quiet Alone

Today's Intention: Date:

What is holding me back?

Celebrations/Concerns: Gratitude:

Opportunities:

"We can easily forgive a child who is afraid of the
dark, the real tragedy of life is when men are afraid
of the light"

                                                    - Plato

My Mantra: Healing Habits:
                                           Water   Movement
                                           Meditation   Sleep
                                           Clean Eating   Visualize
                                           Oral Health   Quiet Alone

Date:

How can I bring more joy into my life?

Gratitude:

Celebrations/Concerns:

Opportunities:

"You have to participate relentlessly in the
manifestation of your own blessings."
~ Elizabeth Gilbert

Healing Habits:

My Mantra:

Water   Movement
Meditation   Sleep
Clean Eating   Visualize
Oral Health   Quiet Alone

Today's Intention: Date:

What can I celebrate today?

Celebrations/Concerns: Gratitude:

Opportunities

"Attention is a tangible measure of love. Whatever
receives our time and attention becomes the center
of gravity, the focus of our life."

- Wayne Muller

My Mantra: Healing Habits:
                                              Water   Movement
                                              Meditation   Sleep
                                              Clean Eating   Visualize
                                              Oral Health   Quiet Alone

Date: Today's Intention:

Do I have what I need?

Gratitude: Celebrations/Concerns:

                                        Opportunities:

'Maybe you are searching among the branches
for what appears only in the roots'
                                ~ Rumi

Healing Habits: My Mantra:

   Water   Movement
   Meditation   Sleep
   Clean Eating   Visualize
   Oral Health   Quiet Alone

Today's Intention: Date

How can I radiate a positive light today?

Celebrations/Concerns: Gratitude:

Opportunities:

"I have decided to stick with love. Hate is too great a
burden to bear."

- Dr. Martin Luther King

My Mantra: Healing Habits:

Water   Movement
Meditation   Sleep
Clean Eating   Visualize
Oral Health   Quiet Alone

Date: Today's Intention:

How can I re-frame my concern to
make it a positive opportunity for
growth?

Gratitude: Celebrations/Concerns:

                                         Opportunities:

"You can't stop the waves, but you can
learn to surf."

                    - Jon Kabat-Zinn

Healing Habits: My Mantra:

   Water   Movement
   Meditation   Sleep
   Clean Eating   Visualize
   Oral Health   Quiet Alone

Today's Intention: Date:

What is my plan for today?

Celebrations/Concerns: Gratitude:

Opportunities:

"In all affairs it's a healthy thing now and then to have a question mark on the things you have long taken for granted."

- Bertrand Russell

My Mantra: Healing Habits:
                                              Water   Movement
                                              Meditation   Sleep
                                              Clean Eating   Visualize
                                              Oral Health   Quiet Alone

Date: Today's Intention:

How can I be of service to others
within my community?

Gratitude: Celebrations/Concerns:

                                   Opportunities:

"Man needs to choose, not just accept his
destiny."
                        - Paulo Coelho

Healing Habits: My Mantra:

   Water   Movement
   Meditation   Sleep
   Clean Eating   Visualize
   Oral Health   Quiet Alone

Today's Intention: Date

What does the brave side of me look like?

Celebrations/Concerns: Gratitude:

Opportunities:

"I live love. I am made of infinite love. I choose love in
each moment."

- Amy Leigh Mercree

My Mantra: Healing Habits:

Water   Movement
Meditation   Sleep
Clean Eating   Visualize
Oral Health   Quiet Alone

What would my life be like if I were not afraid?

Gratitude:

Celebrations/Concerns:

Opportunities:

"You can take no credit for beautiful at sixteen. But, if you are beautiful at sixty, it will be your soul's own doing."
~ Marie Stopes

Healing Habits:

My Mantra:

Water   Movement
Meditation   Sleep
Clean Eating   Visualize
Oral Health   Quiet Alone

Today's Intention: Date:

How can I invite love in my life today?

Celebrations/Concerns: Gratitude:

Opportunities:

"What is a loving heart? A loving heart is sensitive to
the whole of life, to all persons, a loving heart does
not harden itself to any person or thing."
                                        - Anthony de Mello

My Mantra: Healing Habits:
                                        Water   Movement
                                        Meditation   Sleep
                                        Clean Eating   Visualize
                                        Oral Health   Quiet Alone

Date: Today's Intention:

Today I am capable of . . .

Gratitude: Celebrations/Concerns:

                                         Opportunities:

"I never wanted to be a martyr-even for
love. I don't want to die for love. I want to
live for it."

                        - Kamand Kojouri

Healing Habits: My Mantra:

   Water   Movement
   Meditation   Sleep
   Clean Eating   Visualize
   Oral Health   Quiet Alone

Today's Intention: Date:

Where will I find love today?

Celebrations/Concerns: Gratitude:

Opportunities:

"Don't blame a clown for acting like a clown. Ask
yourself why you keep going to the circus."
                                                    ~ Dan Nielsen

My Mantra: Healing Habits:
                                           Water   Movement
                                           Meditation   Sleep
                                           Clean Eating   Visualize
                                           Oral Health   Quiet Alone

What would I look like if I recognized that I am a Being of light and love?

Gratitude:

Celebrations/Concerns:

Opportunities:

"Love is what we are born with. Fear is what we learn. The spiritual journey is the unlearning of fear and prejudices and the acceptance of love back in our hearts. Love is the essential reality and our purpose on earth."

~ Marianne Williamson

Healing Habits:

Water   Movement
Meditation   Sleep
Clean Eating   Visualize
Oral Health   Quiet Alone

My Mantra:

Today's Intention: Date:

I am capable of doing hard things.

Celebrations/Concerns: Gratitude:

Opportunities

"Undoubtedly, we become what we envision."
                                                    - Claude M. Bristol

My Mantra: Healing Habits:
                                                      Water   Movement
                                                      Meditation   Sleep
                                                      Clean Eating   Visualize
                                                      Oral Health   Quiet Alone

Date: Today's Intention:

Dear future me . . .

Gratitude: Celebrations/Concerns:

                                         Opportunities:

"Our life changes the moment we choose love
over hate."
                          - Avijeet Das

Healing Habits: My Mantra:

   Water   Movement
   Meditation   Sleep
   Clean Eating   Visualize
   Oral Health   Quiet Alone

Today's Intention: Date:

What can I let go of to heal a past hurt?

Celebrations/Concerns: Gratitude:

Opportunities:

'When writing the story of your life, don't let
anyone else hold the pen."
                                        - Harly Davidson Ad

My Mantra: Healing Habits:
                                                       Water   Movement
                                                       Meditation   Sleep
                                                       Clean Eating   Visualize
                                                       Oral Health   Quiet Alone

Date: Today's Intention:

I am enough just the way I am today.

Gratitude:

Celebrations/Concerns:

Opportunities:

"Children are happy because they don't have a file in their minds called "All the Things That Could Go Wrong."
— Marianne Williamson

Healing Habits:

   Water   Movement
   Meditation   Sleep
   Clean Eating Visualize
   Oral Health   Quiet Alone

My Mantra:

Today's Intention: Date:

What is one thing I've always wanted to do but not
yet tried?

Celebrations/Concerns: Gratitude:

Opportunities:

"I must not fear. Fear is the mind-killer. Fear is the
little death that brings total obliteration. I will face my
fear. I will permit it to pass over me and through me.
And when it has gone past, I will turn the inner eye to
see its path. Where the fear has gone, there will be
nothing. Only I will remain."

                                                          Frank Herbert

My Mantra: Healing Habits:
                                                Water   Movement
                                                Meditation   Sleep
                                                Clean Eating   Visualize
                                                Oral Health   Quiet Alone

Date: Today's Intention:

One way I will shine today is . . .

Gratitude: Celebrations/Concerns:

                                         Opportunities:

"Every day we are engaged in a miracle which we
don't even recognize: a blue sky, white clouds, green
leaves, the black, curious eyes of a child-our own
two eyes. All is a miracle."
                              - Thich Nhat Hanh

Healing Habits: My Mantra:

   Water   Movement
   Meditation   Sleep
   Clean Eating   Visualize
   Oral Health   Quiet Alone

Today's Intention: Date:

I am able to access compassion best when:

Celebrations/Concerns: Gratitude:

Opportunities:

                                    "The degree to which you love yourself will determine
                                    your ability to love another person, who will be
                                    reflecting back to you many of your own personality
                                    traits and qualities."

                                                              - Sanaya Roman

My Mantra: Healing Habits:
                                        Water   Movement
                                        Meditation   Sleep
                                        Clean Eating   Visualize
                                        Oral Health   Quiet Alone

Date: Today's Intention:

Do I live fully within my own set of values?

Gratitude: Celebrations/Concerns:

                                   Opportunities:

"The day you plant the seed, is not the day you eat the
fruit."
                        - Fabienne Fredrickson

Healing Habits: My Mantra:

   Water   Movement
   Meditation   Sleep
   Clean Eating   Visualize
   Oral Health   Quiet Alone

End of Month Check In

1. How do you feel physically? What needs attention? What has improved?

2. What is your level of self-compassion? What can you do to support deeper self-compassion? What is working right now? What needs focus?

3. What is your level of connection to yourself and others? Can you be of service to others in a positive manner? What is working? What needs focus?

Changing Habits

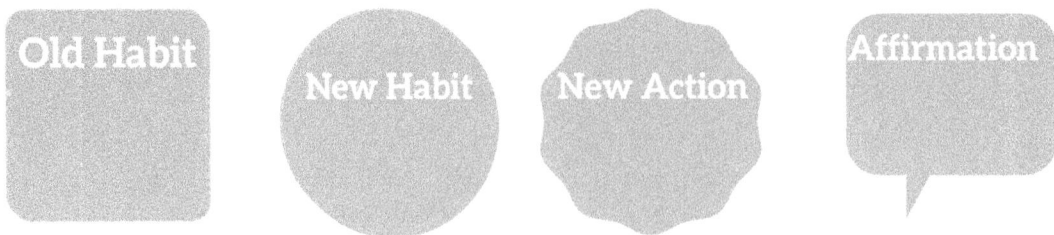

Old Habit

New Habit

New Action

Affirmation

How do I feel?

Love / Safety   Fear / Unsafe

What do I need? Is it safe to process this now?

- What is the base feeling?
- Am I enraged, afraid, blaming, judging?
- Is this feeling coming from love or fear?

- What is the fear?
- Am I afraid of losing something dear?
- Am I afraid of not having enough?
- Am I afraid of what life will look like after this?

- Am I thinking clearly?
- Is there another way to look at this situation?
- Do I have reasonable expectations?
- Is my assertion true?

- What are the possibilities?
- Is there a particular outcome that I am hoping for?
- Can I feel safe if what I want to happen does not?

Love Your Body

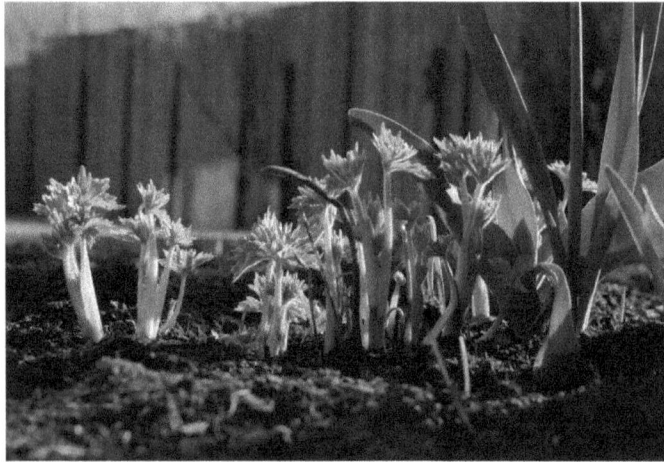

"Doctors won't make you healthy. Nutritionists won't make you slim. Teachers won't make you smart. Gurus won't make you calm. Mentors won't make you rich. Trainers won't make you fit. Ultimately, you have to take responsibility. Save yourself."

~ Naval Ravikant

Book: *I Quit Sugar* by Sarah Wilson

"Yes, I have overcome a lot."

My journey through a medical morass is the genesis of this book. I was morbidly obese for nearly 20 years. There is such shame and guilt in that statement. I had been an active single mother who spent most of her time outdoors with her kid's biking, skiing, hiking, or swimming. My minors in college had been physical education and outdoor education as a nod to a lifetime of great health. A tragic auto accident in 1998 resulted in a severe traumatic head injury and a profound back injury, which involved 18 grueling months of epidural steroid injections, which, in turn, changed my body and life irrevocably. In the aftermath, I gained over 100 lbs, which caused a surge in related medical complications. Even with redoubled efforts to lose weight, I remained obese. Predictably, a cavalcade of other health challenges ganged up in the form of a stroke, another back surgery, and the dreaded colon cancer. I struggled with a medical syndrome that seemed interminable.

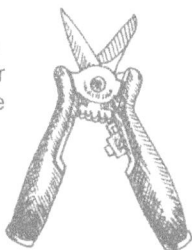

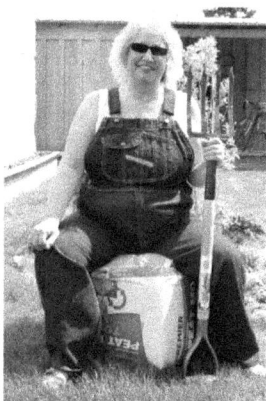

I found a breakthrough in the form of a new approach to healthfulness that focused on reversing systemic inflammation. An inflamed body will hold onto weight and put all its energy into fighting the inflammation, causing weight loss efforts to fail. As I omitted the many foods that my body reacted to, the weight began to finally drop off. My body, once given the chance, started to heal itself. I learned how food affects my body, mind, and soul, and I continue to observe this diet today. While I'm not quite to the "I LOVE my body" stage, I am grateful that I have healed so many diseases and am thriving.

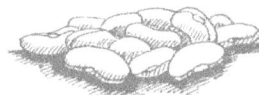

If you have the opportunity, get your medical DNA tested, it can tell you so much about your health. If you have had a miscarriage, or are just starting your family, please ask your doctor to check your MTHFR gene BEFORE you starting taking prenatal vitamins. Your body cannot utilize FOLIC ACID, a chemical version of the B vitamin Folate.

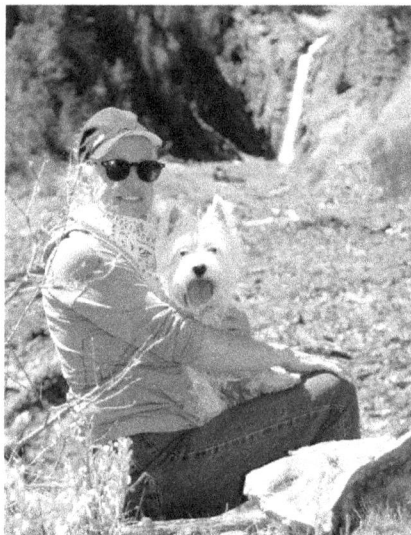

The overriding point here is that I had to challenge and discard core beliefs about food to claim my own well-being. A central theme in this book is the need to do exactly that to become the self-sustaining people we are designed to be. Yes, I have overcome a lot. My life is a testimony that you can do the same. We each have the tools that we need to achieve these personal victories, and journaling is the tool that can uncover the issues as well as intimate their solutions.

Here is the question: Will you live in fear, or will you live in love? I choose love. I invite you to do the same.

Date:

Today's Intention:

Who am I physically? How would I describe my physical health to others?

Gratitude:

Celebrations/Concerns:

Opportunities:

"There are different levels of healing. There is a biological level, an emotional level, a mental level, and, depending on what language you use, a spiritual level."
— Dr. Michael Learner

Healing Habits:

Water   Movement
Meditation   Sleep
Clean Eating   Visualize
Oral Health   Quiet Alone

My Mantra:

Today's Intention: Date:

What do I need to support my best health?

Celebrations/Concerns: Gratitude:

Opportunities:

"Meet me in the middle of your story when the soul is
worn but wise."

- Angie. Weiland Crosby

My Mantra: Healing Habits:

Water   Movement
Meditation   Sleep
Clean Eating   Visualize
Oral Health   Quiet Alone

Date: _____ Today's Intention:

How can I be of service others?

Gratitude: Celebrations/Concerns:

Opportunities:

"Wounds that we inflict upon ourselves are the most
difficult to heal".
                              - Theodor Reik

Healing Habits: My Mantra:

Water   Movement
Meditation   Sleep
Clean Eating   Visualize
Oral Health   Quiet Alone

Today's Intention: Date:

How do I feel about my body?

Celebrations/Concerns: Gratitude:

Opportunities:

"In China, the patient is responsible for helping to
prevent illness and maintain health. Try to center
yourself and feel balanced."
                                              - Dr. David Eisenberg

My Mantra: Healing Habits:
                                              Water   Movement
                                              Meditation   Sleep
                                              Clean Eating   Visualize
                                              Oral Health   Quiet Alone

Date:

My body is . . . .

Gratitude:

Celebrations/Concerns:

Opportunities:

"You cannot put the same shoe on every foot."
- Publilius Syrus

Healing Habits:

Water   Movement
Meditation   Sleep
Clean Eating   Visualize
Oral Health   Quiet Alone

My Mantra:

Today's Intention: Date:

What makes you beautiful?

Celebrations/Concerns: Gratitude:

Opportunities:

"See if you can catch yourself complaining in either
speech or thought about a situation you find yourself
in, what other people do or say, your surroundings,
your life situation, even the weather. To complain is
always non-acceptance of what is. It invariably carries
an unconscious negative charge. When you complain, you
make yourself a victim. Leave the situation or accept
it. All else is madness."

                                                          - Eckhart Tolle

My Mantra: Healing Habits:
                                                    Water   Movement
                                                    Meditation   Sleep
                                                    Clean Eating   Visualize
                                                    Oral Health   Quiet Alone

Date: Today's Intention:

What part of my body would i like to
change?

Gratitude: Celebrations/Concerns:

                                         Opportunities:

"Health is not a condition of matter but of mind."
                          - Mary Baker Eddy

Healing Habits: My Mantra:

    Water   Movement
    Meditation   Sleep
    Clean Eating   Visualize
    Oral Health   Quiet Alone

Today's Intention: Date:

How can I best nourish and heal my body?

Celebrations/Concerns: Gratitude:

Opportunities:

"Tomorrow, you promise yourself, will be different, yet
tomorrow is too often a repetition of today."
                                                      - James T. McCay

My Mantra: Healing Habits:
                                             Water   Movement
                                             Meditation   Sleep
                                             Clean Eating   Visualize
                                             Oral Health   Quiet Alone

Date: _____   Today's Intention: _____

What does my body need to feel safe?

Gratitude: Celebrations/Concerns:

                                          Opportunities:

"You can still change your story."
          - Don Miguel Ruiz

Healing Habits: My Mantra:

    Water   Movement
    Meditation   Sleep
    Clean Eating   Visualize
    Oral Health   Quiet Alone

Today's Intention: Date:

How do i take care of my body?

Celebrations/Concerns: Gratitude:

Opportunities:

"Every thought you have travels through your biological system and activates a physiological response. Some thoughts, like fear, are like depth charges, causing a reaction throughout your body, a loving thought can relax your entire body. Some thoughts are more subtle, and still others are unconscious."

- Carolyn Myss

My Mantra: Healing Habits:

Water   Movement
Meditation   Sleep
Clean Eating   Visualize
Oral Health   Quiet Alone

What do my daily self-care habits say
about how I feel about my body?

Gratitude:

Celebrations/Concerns:

Opportunities:

"Am I willing to give up what I have in order to be what
I am not yet?"

- Mary Caroline Richards

Healing Habits:

    Water   Movement
    Meditation   Sleep
    Clean Eating   Visualize
    Oral Health   Quiet Alone

My Mantra:

Today's Intention: Date

Do my daily health care habits reflect the way I want to
take care of my body? If yes, explain. If no, what small
steps can I take to change that?

Celebrations/Concerns: Gratitude:

Opportunities:

"Before healing others, heal yourself."
- Gambian Proverb

My Mantra: Healing Habits:
                                             Water   Movement
                                             Meditation   Sleep
                                             Clean Eating   Visualize
                                             Oral Health   Quiet Alone

Do I drink enough water daily to clean out accumulated toxins?

Gratitude:

Celebrations/Concerns:

Opportunities:

"Get into the habit of asking yourself, 'Does this support the life I am trying to create'?"
- Conscious Magazine

Healing Habits:

Water   Movement
Meditation   Sleep
Clean Eating   Visualize
Oral Health   Quiet Alone

My Mantra:

Today's Intention: Date:

Do i tend to my oral health daily by brushing my teeth and
flossing?

Celebrations/Concerns: Gratitude:

Opportunities:

"I believe that the greatest gift you can give your family
and the world is a healthy you."

- Joyce Meyer

My Mantra: Healing Habits:
                                         Water   Movement
                                         Meditation   Sleep
                                         Clean Eating   Visualize
                                         Oral Health   Quiet Alone

Date: Today's Intention:

How do I move my body daily?

Gratitude: Celebrations/Concerns:

                                         Opportunities:

"Moderation. Small helpings. Sample a little bit of
everything. These are the secrets of happiness and
good health."

                              - Julia Child

Healing Habits: My Mantra:

    Water   Movement
    Meditation   Sleep
    Clean Eating   Visualize
    Oral Health   Quiet Alone

Today's Intention: Date

Do i sleep well? Describe my typical sleep experience.

Celebrations/Concerns: Gratitude:

Opportunities:

"The root of all desire is the one desire to come home,
to be at peace."

- Jean Klein

My Mantra: Healing Habits:

Water   Movement
Meditation   Sleep
Clean Eating   Visualize
Oral Health   Quiet Alone

Date: Today's Intention:

What is my favorite thing about my
sleeping space?

Gratitude: Celebrations/Concerns:

                                Opportunities:

"Nobody can be in good health if he does not have all
the time fresh air, sunshine and good water."
          - Flying Hawk (Native American Proverb)

Healing Habits: My Mantra:

    Water   Movement
    Meditation   Sleep
    Clean Eating Visualize
    Oral Health Quiet Alone

Today's Intention: Date:

Do i sleep enough to wake up looking forward to each
new day?

Celebrations/Concerns: Gratitude:

Opportunities:

"Life is like a tree and its root is consciousness.
Therefore, once we tend the root, the tree as a whole
will be healthy."

- Deepak Chopra

My Mantra: Healing Habits:

                                                   Water   Movement
                                                   Meditation   Sleep
                                                   Clean Eating   Visualize
                                                   Oral Health   Quiet Alone

Date: _____

Today's Intention: _____

Do I feel good about how much I accomplish each day?

Gratitude:

Celebrations/Concerns:

Opportunities:

"Sickness: nature's vengeance for violating her laws."
- Charles Simmons

Healing Habits:

Water   Movement
Meditation   Sleep
Clean Eating   Visualize
Oral Health   Quiet Alone

My Mantra:

Today's Intention: Date:

How did I love spending my free time as a child? How can I incorporate that into today?

Celebrations/Concerns: Gratitude:

Opportunities:

"I am not afraid of my truth anymore, and I will not omit pieces of myself to make you more comfortable."

- Alexandra Elle

My Mantra: Healing Habits:

Water	Movement
Meditation	Sleep
Clean Eating	Visualize
Oral Health	Quiet Alone

Today's Intention:

What can I do to reduce toxins in my daily
life?

Gratitude: Celebrations/Concerns:

                                        Opportunities:

"You must do the thing you think you cannot do."
                        ~ Eleanor Roosevelt

Healing Habits: My Mantra:

    Water   Movement
    Meditation   Sleep
    Clean Eating   Visualize
    Oral Health   Quiet Alone

Today's Intention: Date:

Do i have pain in my body? How much? Where? When is it present?

Celebrations/Concerns: Gratitude:

Opportunities:

"If you can dream it, you can do it."
~ Walt Disney

My Mantra: Healing Habits:
                                                   Water   Movement
                                                   Meditation   Sleep
                                                   Clean Eating   Visualize
                                                   Oral Health   Quiet Alone

Date: Today's Intention:

Do I have pain in my body? How much?
Where? When is it present?

Gratitude: Celebrations/Concerns:

                                         Opportunities:

.

"If you can dream it, you can do it."
                      ~ Walt Disney

Healing Habits: My Mantra:

   Water   Movement
   Meditation   Sleep
   Clean Eating   Visualize
   Oral Health   Quiet Alone

Today's Intention: Date:

What can I change in my diet to improve my life?

Celebrations/Concerns: Gratitude:

Opportunities:

"Find out who you are, then do it on purpose."
- Dolly Parton

My Mantra: Healing Habits:

Water	Movement
Meditation	Sleep
Clean Eating	Visualize
Oral Health	Quiet Alone

Date:

How can I incorporate more fruit into my diet?

Gratitude:

Celebrations/Concerns:

Opportunities:

"The wish for healing has always been half of health"
- Lucius Annaeus Seneca

Healing Habits:

My Mantra:

Water   Movement
Meditation   Sleep
Clean Eating   Visualize
Oral Health   Quiet Alone

Today's Intention: Date:

How can I incorporate more fiber into my diet?

Celebrations/Concerns: Gratitude:

Opportunities:

"The greatest of follies is to sacrifice health for any
other kind of happiness."

- Arthur Schopenhauer

My Mantra: Healing Habits:
                                                Water   Movement
                                                Meditation   Sleep
                                                Clean Eating   Visualize
                                                Oral Health   Quiet Alone

Date: Today's Intention

My favorite way to incorporate movement
into my life daily is . . . .

Gratitude: Celebrations/Concerns:

                                         Opportunities:

"What is called genius is the abundance of life and
health."
                    - Henry David Thoreau

Healing Habits: My Mantra:

    Water   Movement
    Meditation   Sleep
    Clean Eating Visualize
    Oral Health   Quiet Alone

Today's Intention: Date:

How can I live my best life exactly as I am today?

Celebrations/Concerns: Gratitude:

Opportunities:

"Sometimes the smallest step in the right direction ends
up being the biggest step our your life, tiptoe if you
must, but take the step"

- Naeem Calloway

My Mantra: Healing Habits:

                                              Water   Movement
                                              Meditation   Sleep
                                              Clean Eating   Visualize
                                              Oral Health   Quiet Alone

End of Month Check In

1. How do you feel physically? What needs attention? What has improved?

2. What is your level of self-compassion? What can you do to support deeper self-compassion? What is working right now? What needs focus?

3. What is your level of connection to yourself and others? Can you be of service to others in a positive manner? What is working? What needs focus?

Changing Habits

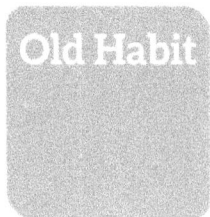

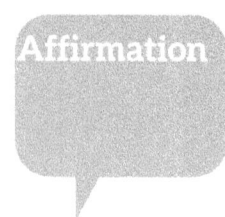

Old Habit

New Habit

New Action

Affirmation

FOOD AND BODY TRACKER

Date _____

Current Eating Plan _____ Days of Consistant Following of plan _____

Intention _____ Goal _____

FOOD INTAKE

Include everything that goes in your mouth. List amount and time of day, note immediate symptoms, delayed symptoms, and overall physical and emotional response to intake.

PHYSICAL ALERTS

Skin Appearance
Gastric Upset
Congestion or Runny Nose
Pain or Inflammation
Gas or Bloating

EMOTIONAL ALERTS

Mood Fluctuation
Grumpiness Meter
Sad / Mad / Depressed
Temper Flair UP
Peaceful and Calm

MOVEMENT

Yoga - Swimming - Biking
Hiking - Running - Walking
Stretching - Aerobic
Breathing Exercises

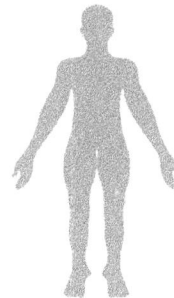

Mindfulness

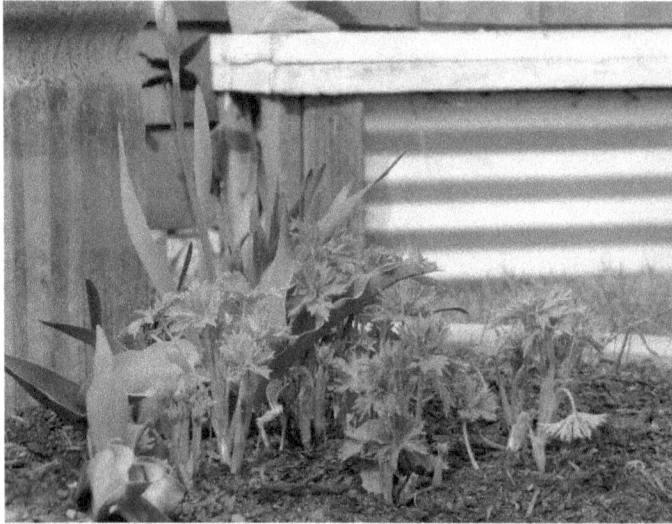

"Mindfulness is simply being aware of what is happening right now without wishing it were different; enjoying the pleasant without holding on when it changes (which it will); being with the unpleasant without fearing it will always be this way (which it won't)."

~ James Baraz

Book: *The Mindful Path to Self-Compassion: Freeing Yourself From Destructive Thoughts and Emotions* by Christopher K Germer

"Journaling is the tool. Mindfulness is the outcome."

Journaling is the tool. Mindfulness is the outcome. They connect and support one another. For me, mindfulness means living in the moment, not guilt-tripping over what already has passed or anxiously tweaking about what might happen in the future. Writing and journaling have gotten me through many difficult moments since I was a girl in elementary school. I've done a lot of journaling to support the process of understanding my body and health. I consider my morning journaling time as "writing to wellness." Writing allows me to stay focused on the moment and not get lost in the "what ifs," simply being here now. As I write these words into my computer right now, I am focused on the sounds of the ticking keyboard, the birds chirping outside, and the happy sound of two chickens quietly clucking over food. For me, that's my reality: the sights and sounds of the day. Being present to the momentary realities in life engenders wellness. That ticking of the keyboard and chirping of the birds, soaking up the sun, and marveling at the blue sky, all yield wellness.

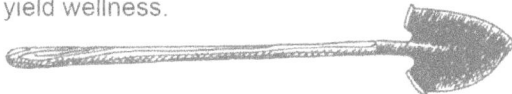

I reestablished my journaling habit earnestly when I got out of the hospital after my cancer surgery, Christmas of 2016. I tracked food, movement, pain, and skin conditions. In fact, I tracked all of my health closely, developing my sense of Self through mindfulness. In some ways, journaling is self-excavation, digging into personal depths to uncover long-overlooked treasures. It's a lot like personal archeology that way.

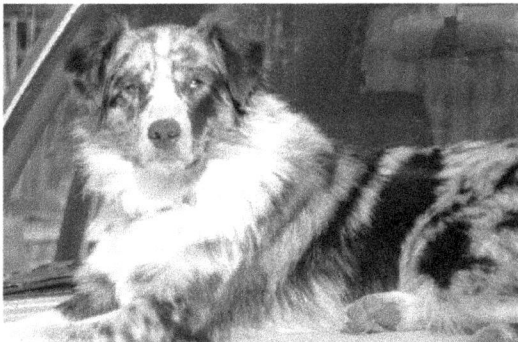

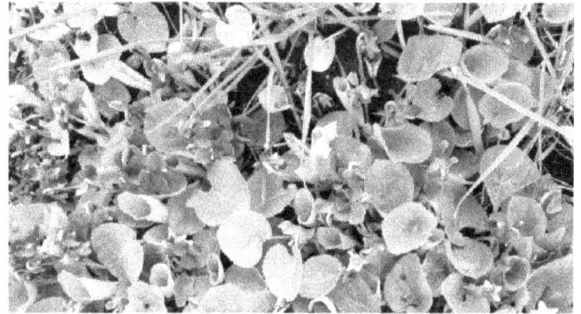

After my cancer surgery, writing each morning and most evenings was therapeutic and helped my trusted healers and me figure out what was truly going on with my body. I know what my limitations and challenges are, and have found creative ways to live fully using various hacks to bypass what I can no longer do.

I have vibrant health within my limitations, and I am so grateful. Remarkably, I am actually quite close to my ideal weight in high school by eating foods closer to their natural state than ever. I have food freedom and live and breathe in the present. I seek balance, and journaling allows me to catch myself before I get out of balance.

Give a listen to the children playing outside, to the birds chirping, to the flowers groping for the sun. As you do, try and realize that you too are part of the magnificently beautiful scenery in life. Through mindfulness, we learn that we, too, belong.

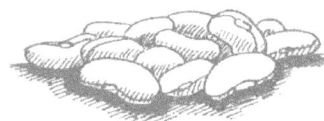

However you choose to describe meditation, it is scientifically proven to be beneficial to body, mind, and soul. Some call it prayer, others call it a quiet time or a time out, others simply practice it without a verbal description. Choose to think deeply and explore your True Self.

Date: Today's Intention:

Who am I right now?

Gratitude:

Celebrations/Concerns:

Opportunities:

"When we are no longer able to change a situation, we are challenged do change ourselves."

- Victor Frankl

Healing Habits:

Water   Movement
Meditation   Sleep
Clean Eating   Visualize
Oral Health   Quiet Alone

My Mantra:

Today's Intention: Date:

What do I want for myself intellectually?

Celebrations/Concerns: Gratitude:

Opportunities:

"One day you'll look back and see that all along you were blooming."

- Morgan Harper Nicoles

My Mantra: Healing Habits:

Water   Movement
Meditation   Sleep
Clean Eating   Visualize
Oral Health   Quiet Alone

Today's Intention:

How can I be of service today?

Gratitude:

Celebrations/Concerns:

Opportunities:

Everything has it's wonders, even darkness, and
silence, and I learn whatever state I may be in, therein
to be content."

- Helen Keller

Healing Habits:

Water   Movement
Meditation   Sleep
Clean Eating   Visualize
Oral Health   Quiet Alone

My Mantra:

Today's Intention: Date:

How do I learn best? Hands-on? Seeing? Reading?
Experiencing? Hearing?

Celebrations/Concerns: Gratitude:

Opportunities:

"They seemed to come suddenly upon happiness as if
they had surprised a butterfly in the woods . . ."
                                    - Edith Wharton

My Mantra: Healing Habits:
                                        Water   Movement
                                        Meditation   Sleep
                                        Clean Eating   Visualize
                                        Oral Health   Quiet Alone

Date: _____

What is my greatest strength?

Gratitude:

Celebrations/Concerns:

Opportunities:

"Everything in life happens according to our time our clock. You may look at some of your friends and think that they're ahead of you. Maybe some of them you feel are behind, but everything happens at it's own pace. They have their own time and clock and so do you. Be patient."

— Jay Shetty

Healing Habits:

Water   Movement
Meditation   Sleep
Clean Eating   Visualize
Oral Health   Quiet Alone

My Mantra:

Today's Intention: Date:

What is a weakness that I would like to address?

Celebrations/Concerns: Gratitude:

Opportunities:

"We repeat what we don't repair."
- Christine Langly Obaugh

My Mantra: Healing Habits:
                                                  Water   Movement
                                                  Meditation   Sleep
                                                  Clean Eating   Visualize
                                                  Oral Health   Quiet Alone

Date: _____

What do I love most about the people i
spend the most time with?

Gratitude:

Celebrations/Concerns:

Opportunities:

"It is you that chooses to linger in resentment, or to
be consumed by anger, or enveloped in grief, or to
release these lower-frequency currents of energy"
                                            - Gary Zukav

Healing Habits:

Water   Movement
Meditation   Sleep
Clean Eating   Visualize
Oral Health   Quiet Alone

My Mantra:

Today's Intention: Date:

What brings me joy?

Celebrations/Concerns: Gratitude:

Opportunities:

"Failures are only failures when we don't learn from
them because when we learn from them they become
lessons."

- Jay Shetty

My Mantra: Healing Habits:

                                          Water   Movement
                                          Meditation   Sleep
                                          Clean Eating   Visualize
                                          Oral Health   Quiet Alone

Date: _____   Today's Intention: _____

Where (location) do you feel the most joy?

Gratitude: Celebrations/Concerns:

                                Opportunities:

"If your path demands you walk through hell, walk as
if you own the place."

                                    - Gaurav Singh

Healing Habits: My Mantra:

Water   Movement
Meditation   Sleep
Clean Eating   Visualize
Oral Health   Quiet Alone

Today's Intention: Date:

What is beautiful around me right now?

Celebrations/Concerns: Gratitude:

Opportunities:

"There is something infinitely healing in the repeated
refrains for nature . . . the assurance that dawn
comes after night and that Spring comes after
Winter."

                                              - Rachel Carson

My Mantra: Healing Habits:

                                                   Water   Movement
                                                   Meditation   Sleep
                                                   Clean Eating   Visualize
                                                   Oral Health   Quiet Alone

Date: Today's Intention:

What brings me peace?

Gratitude: Celebrations/Concerns:

"There is no greater gift you can give or receive than   Opportunities:
to honor your calling. It is why you were born and
how you will become most truly alive."
                              ~ Oprah Winfrey

Healing Habits: My Mantra:

Water   Movement
Meditation   Sleep
Clean Eating   Visualize
Oral Health   Quiet Alone

Today's Intention: Date:

What creates a sense of calm around me?

Celebrations/Concerns: Gratitude:

Opportunities:

"The secret of health for both mind and body is not to
mourn for the past, not to worry about the future,
or not to anticipate troubles, but to live in the present
moment wisely and earnestly." ~ Buddha

My Mantra: Healing Habits:

                                                   Water   Movement
                                                   Meditation   Sleep
                                                   Clean Eating   Visualize
                                                   Oral Health   Quiet Alone

Date: _____

Are healing and excellent health top
priorities for me?

Gratitude: Celebrations/Concerns:

                              Opportunities:

"Having a beautiful soul doesn't mean you're pure and
spotless, it's being able to consistently come back with
a heart of love and compassion despite your
imperfection as a human being."
                                    - Unknown

Healing Habits: My Mantra:

  Water   Movement
  Meditation   Sleep
  Clean Eating Visualize
  Oral Health Quiet Alone

Today's Intention: Date:

What do i have in my life today that brings me joy?

Celebrations/Concerns: Gratitude:

Opportunities:

"The more you understand yourself, the more silence
there is, the healthier you are."

- Maxime Lagace

My Mantra: Healing Habits:

Water   Movement
Meditation   Sleep
Clean Eating   Visualize
Oral Health   Quiet Alone

Date: _____   Today's Intention: _____

What opportunities will I seek today?

Gratitude: Celebrations/Concerns:

                                    Opportunities:

"There is no education like adversity."
                    - Walt Disney

Healing Habits: My Mantra:

   Water   Movement
   Meditation   Sleep
   Clean Eating Visualize
   Oral Health Quiet Alone

Today's Intention: Date:

How can i feel the best in my body today?

Celebrations/Concerns: Gratitude:

Opportunities:

"Decide what kind of life you actually want. Then . . .
say no to everything that isn't that"

                                          - Bryan Svanak

My Mantra: Healing Habits:
                                          Water   Movement
                                          Meditation   Sleep
                                          Clean Eating   Visualize
                                          Oral Health   Quiet Alone

Date

Describe my favorite evening rituals that support a better night's sleep?

Gratitude:

Celebrations/Concerns:

Opportunities:

"Your body hears everything your mind says."
- Naomi Judd

Healing Habits:

Water   Movement
Meditation   Sleep
Clean Eating   Visualize
Oral Health   Quiet Alone

My Mantra:

Today's Intention: Date:

What can i do to make another person smile today?

Celebrations/Concerns: Gratitude:

Opportunities:

"Health is a large word It embraces not the body only,
but the mind and spirit as well; . . . and not today's pain
or pleasure alone, but the whole being and outlook of a
man."

- James H. West

My Mantra: Healing Habits:
                                                    Water   Movement
                                                    Meditation   Sleep
                                                    Clean Eating   Visualize
                                                    Oral Health   Quiet Alone

How can I best take care of myself
today?

Gratitude:

Celebrations/Concerns:

Opportunities:

"Health is the first muse, comprising the magical
benefits of air, landscape, and bodily exercise on the
mind."

- Ralph Waldo Emerson

Healing Habits:

Water   Movement
Meditation   Sleep
Clean Eating   Visualize
Oral Health   Quiet Alone

My Mantra:

Today's Intention: Date:

What can I do outside today to support optimal health?

Celebrations/Concerns: Gratitude:

Opportunities:

"When emotion waves come crashing against your soul,
stay calm. Just like the ocean waves, they ebb and
flow. Stay centered. Let the waves wash through you.
If the ocean can calm itself, so can you."
                                          - Musings of a Mystic

My Mantra: Healing Habits:
                                       Water   Movement
                                       Meditation   Sleep
                                       Clean Eating   Visualize
                                       Oral Health   Quiet Alone

How can i bring rest and relaxation into
my day today?

Gratitude: Celebrations/Concerns:

                                              Opportunities:

"There is one consolation in being sick, and that is the
possibility that you may recover to a better state
than you were ever in before."
                                    - Henry David Thoreau

Healing Habits: My Mantra:

   Water   Movement
   Meditation   Sleep
   Clean Eating   Visualize
   Oral Health   Quiet Alone

Today's Intention: Date:

Is my life well balanced? What can I do today to restore
balance?

Celebrations/Concerns: Gratitude:

Opportunities:

"Health is a vehicle, not a destination."
- Joshua Fields Millburn

My Mantra: Healing Habits:
                                       Water   Movement
                                       Meditation   Sleep
                                       Clean Eating   Visualize
                                       Oral Health   Quiet Alone

Today's Intention:

What can I do to add movement to my day?

Gratitude:

Celebrations/Concerns:

Opportunities:

"The mindfulness revolution is not quite as dramatic as the moon shot or the civil rights movement, but I believe, in the long run, it can have just as great an impact."

— Tim Ryan

Healing Habits:

Water
Meditation
Clean Eating
Oral Health

Movement
Sleep
Visualize
Quiet Alone

My Mantra:

Today's Intention: Date:

How can i connect more deeply to today?

Celebrations/Concerns: Gratitude:

Opportunities:

"The mind and body are not separate units, but one
integrated system. How we act and what we think, eat,
and feel are all related to our health. Physicians should
be capable of teaching this behavior to patients."
                                                    - Bernie Siegel

My Mantra: Healing Habits:

                                                    Water   Movement
                                                    Meditation   Sleep
                                                    Clean Eating   Visualize
                                                    Oral Health   Quiet Alone

Can I incorporate compassion today?

Gratitude: Celebrations/Concerns:

                                              Opportunities:

"There is no diet that will do what eating healthy does."
                                        - Unknown

Healing Habits: My Mantra:

    Water   Movement
    Meditation   Sleep
    Clean Eating   Visualize
    Oral Health   Quiet Alone

Today's Intention: Date:

Today I will remain mindful

Celebrations/Concerns: Gratitude:

Opportunities:

"There is only one success: to spend your life in your own way"

- Chrisopher Morley

My Mantra: Healing Habits:
                                                Water   Movement
                                                Meditation   Sleep
                                                Clean Eating   Visualize
                                                Oral Health   Quiet Alone

Date: Today's Intention:

What is one thing I can do today to fulfill
my purpose?

Gratitude:

Celebrations/Concerns:

Opportunities:

"I really love yoga. I love the mindfulness of it, where
not only are you exercising your body, but you're also
building that mind/body connection as far as being
aware of every movement - what your body's doing,
how your body's feeling"

　　　　　　　　　　　- Miranda Rae Mayo

Healing Habits:

My Mantra:

Water   Movement
Meditation   Sleep
Clean Eating   Visualize
Oral Health   Quiet Alone

128

Today's Intention: Date:

How can i share hope today?

Celebrations/Concerns: Gratitude:

Opportunities:

"Walk as if you are kissing the Earth with your feet."
- Thich Nhat Hanh

My Mantra: Healing Habits:
                                                    Water   Movement
                                                    Meditation   Sleep
                                                    Clean Eating   Visualize
                                                    Oral Health   Quiet Alone

Today I will be aware of wonder.

Gratitude:

Celebrations/Concerns:

Opportunities:

"The most fundamental aggression to ourselves, the most fundamental harm we can do to ourselves, is to remain ignorant by not having the courage and the respect to look at ourselves honestly and gently."
						- Pema Chodron

Healing Habits:

Water   Movement
Meditation   Sleep
Clean Eating   Visualize
Oral Health   Quiet Alone

My Mantra:

Today's Intention: Date:

What is a recent happy thought?

Celebrations/Concerns: Gratitude:

Opportunities:

"Mindfulness has helped me succeed in almost every
dimension of my life. By stopping regularly to look
inward and become aware of my mental state, i stay
connected to the source of my actions and thoughts
and can guide them with considerably more intention."
                                            - Dustin Moskovitz

My Mantra: Healing Habits:

                                        Water   Movement
                                        Meditation   Sleep
                                        Clean Eating   Visualize
                                        Oral Health   Quiet Alone

One way I will shine today is . . . .

Gratitude:

Celebrations/Concerns:

Opportunities.

"Every day we are engaged in a miracle which we
don't even recognize: a blue sky, white clouds, green
leaves, the black, curious eyes of a child-our own two
eyes. All is a miracle."

- Thich Nhat Hanh

Healing Habits:

Water   Movement
Meditation   Sleep
Clean Eating   Visualize
Oral Health   Quiet Alone

My Mantra:

End of Month Check In

1. How do you feel physically? What needs attention? What has improved?

2. What is your level of self-compassion? What can you do to support deeper self-compassion? What is working right now? What needs focus?

3. What is your level of connection to yourself and others? Can you be of service to others in a positive manner? What is working? What needs focus?

Changing Habits

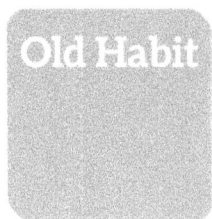

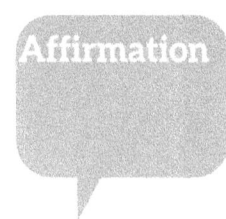

Old Habit

New Habit

New Action

Affirmation

Mindfulness

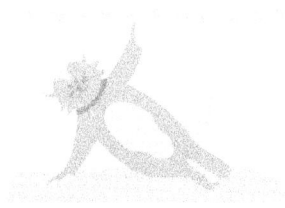

QUIET TIME AND SPACE   SET A TIMER

FIND A COMFORTABLE   TAKE A DEEP CLEANSING
POSITION   BREATH

Intention for this Meditation Session

Pay attention to your breath. Choose a breathing pattern and stick with it for 8 rounds.

- Ask a question to your True Self
- Ask for clarity.
- Am I comfortable with the way my life has been going?
- Am I in balance? Physically, Emotionally, Socially, Intellectually and Spiritually?

- Remain physically still and in place.
- Focus on your breath.
- If your mind wanders consider "weed" or "seed," and 'let go or consider.'

Compassion

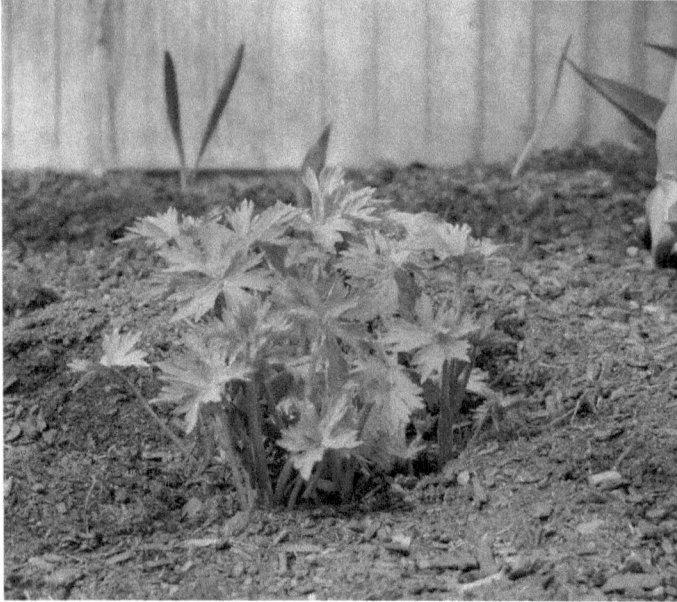

""Joy is not a constant, It comes to us in moments - often ordinary moments. Sometimes we miss out on the bursts of joy because we're too busy chasing down the extraordinary moments. Other times we're so afraid of the dark we don't dare let ourselves enjoy the light. A joyful life is not a floodlight of joy. That would eventually become unbearable. I believe a joyful life is made up of joyful moments gracefully strung together by trust, gratitude, and inspiration."

~Brene' Brown

Book: *Radical Compassion* by Tara Brach

"What are your feelings about self-love?"

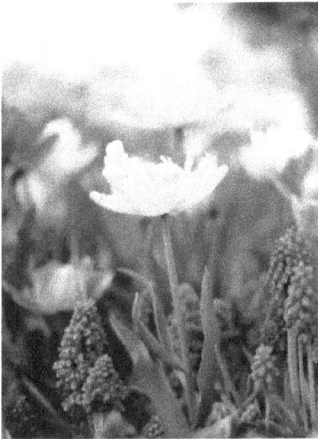

When I was 8 years old, I had a pivotal childhood experience that has been with me all my life. As a child in a very conservative church, we were told that it was a sin to love yourself, though the memory verse was, "Love your neighbor as yourself." Even as a young child, this didn't make sense. How sad to receive such a convoluted message as a child! I now know that becoming my Best Self cannot happen unless I love myself by putting the hard work in to become exactly that. By choosing love and letting go of fear, I choose self-compassion, which gets stretched to the limit with chronic illness and multiple health challenges. I had to see value in myself to move forward.

Having a clearly defined purpose has helped. During the time when I thought my life was coming to an end, I prepared to have a healthy end-of-life experience. I journaled at least once a day, meditated daily, looking deeply at the shape and textures of my life. I considered where I had been and what I had experienced to make the woman I am today.

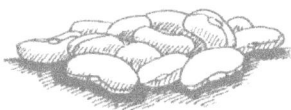

One of the most important factors in connection is communication - have conversations in person, eye to eye for truly effective communication - gauging how the person you are speaking to is RECEIVING your message is an essential part of effective communication. Texts and emails often create more confusion and conflict.

Rather than focusing on the gloom and doom that were very real in my life, I sought out the rainbows that promised a better tomorrow. Slowly, a sense of self-purpose gained momentum. Through self-love, I began to internalize my real worth as a strong woman of voice, one that I am sharing with you right now. However, I really had to stick with it, and journaling has been the tool of that discovery and maintenance. I am still working on accepting my humanity, that I err, that I have maladaptive behaviors that pop up like old reruns here and there, but each day feels a little closer to being my own best friend. Journaling has introduced me to myself.

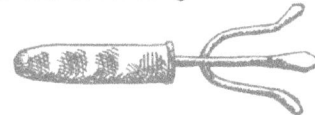

What are your feelings about self-love? Are you comfortable with yourself? Can you step back and observe your thoughts, emotions, and experiences and learn from them? Have you incorporated gratitude into your life to support healing and invite grace? This is your opportunity to show yourself the same grace that you would offer a dearly loved member of family or circle of friends. Yes, you are worthy of self-love. I would encourage you to begin taking steps along this path. Doing so will empower you to be your most brilliant Self.

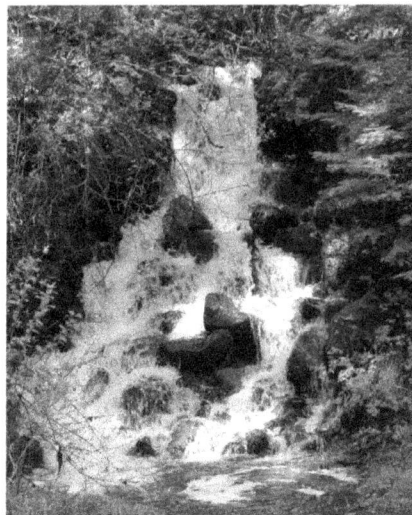

Date: _____

Who am I around others? Are my interactions positive and consistent across all settings?

Gratitude:

Celebrations/Concerns:

Opportunities:

"Cherish that which is within you"
                - Chuang-Tzu

Healing Habits:

Water   Movement
Meditation   Sleep
Clean Eating   Visualize
Oral Health   Quiet Alone

My Mantra:

Today's Intention: Date:

What do I want in a friendship?

Celebrations/Concerns: Gratitude:

Opportunities:

"I think the reward for conformity is that everyone likes you except yourself."

- Rita Mae Brown

My Mantra: Healing Habits:

Water   Movement
Meditation   Sleep
Clean Eating   Visualize
Oral Health   Quiet Alone

How can I be of service using compassion as a guide?

Gratitude:

Celebrations/Concerns:

Opportunities:

"Friendship with oneself is all-important because without one cannot be friends with anyone else in the world."

- Eleanor Roosevelt

Healing Habits:

Water   Movement
Meditation   Sleep
Clean Eating   Visualize
Oral Health   Quiet Alone

My Mantra:

Today's Intention: Date:

What kind of friend am I?

Celebrations/Concerns: Gratitude:

Opportunities:

"You have to live with yourself at least reasonably well before you are able to live with a mate. There must be certain self-esteem before you can expect that other people will value you highly."

- Theodor Reik

My Mantra: Healing Habits:
                                                Water   Movement
                                                Meditation   Sleep
                                                Clean Eating   Visualize
                                                Oral Health   Quiet Alone

Date:

Which strengths will I draw upon today?

Gratitude:

Celebrations/Concerns:

Opportunities:

"If you want to experience love, you have to start by loving yourself."

- Swami Muktananda

Healing Habits:

Water   Movement
Meditation   Sleep
Clean Eating   Visualize
Oral Health   Quiet Alone

My Mantra:

Today's Intention: Date:

How do i feel about those who i spend the most time with? Do they bring out the positive energy in me?

Celebrations/Concerns: Gratitude:

Opportunities:

"Do your own thing and don't care if they don't like it"
- Tina Fey

My Mantra:

Healing Habits:

Water   Movement
Meditation   Sleep
Clean Eating   Visualize
Oral Health   Quiet Alone

Date

How can I give myself grace today?

Gratitude:

Celebrations/Concerns:

Opportunities:

"Life is short, but there is always time for compassion."
- Ralph Waldo Emmerson

Healing Habits:

Water   Movement
Meditation   Sleep
Clean Eating   Visualize
Oral Health   Quiet Alone

My Mantra:

Today's Intention: Date:

Can i share compassion today?

Celebrations/Concerns: Gratitude:

Opportunities:

"Self-acceptance comes from meeting life's challenges
vigorously. Don't numb yourself to your trials and
difficulties, nor build mental walls to exclude pain from
your life. You will find peace not by trying to escape your
problems, but by confronting them courageously. You will
find peace not in denial, but in victory."
                                            - J. Donald Walters

My Mantra: Healing Habits:
                                          Water   Movement
                                          Meditation   Sleep
                                          Clean Eating   Visualize
                                          Oral Health   Quiet Alone

Date:

What does self-compassion mean to me?

Gratitude:

Celebrations/Concerns:

Opportunities:

"When a woman becomes her own best friend, life is easier."

- Diane Von Furstenberg

Healing Habits:

Water   Movement
Meditation   Sleep
Clean Eating   Visualize
Oral Health   Quiet Alone

My Mantra:

Today's Intention: _____ Date: _____

At what point in life have I felt most loved and
supported?

Celebrations/Concerns: Gratitude:

Opportunities:

"There is a vitality, a life force, an energy, a quickening,
that is translated through you into action, and because
there is only one of you in all time, this expression is
unique. And if you block it, it will never exist through any
other medium and will be lost."

- Martha Graham

My Mantra: _____

Healing Habits:

Water	Movement
Meditation	Sleep
Clean Eating	Visualize
Oral Health	Quiet Alone

147

What inspires compassion towards others?

Gratitude:

Celebrations/Concerns:

Opportunities:

"The best doctor gives the least medicine."
- Benjamin Franklin

Healing Habits:

Water   Movement
Meditation   Sleep
Clean Eating   Visualize
Oral Health   Quiet Alone

My Mantra

Today's Intention: Date:

Self-love is:

Celebrations/Concerns: Gratitude:

Opportunities:

"To be beautiful means to be yourself. You don't need to
be accepted by others. You need to accept yourself."
                                                    - Thich Nhat Hanh

My Mantra: Healing Habits:
                                            Water   Movement
                                            Meditation   Sleep
                                            Clean Eating   Visualize
                                            Oral Health   Quiet Alone

How does self-compassion help me reach my personal goals?

Gratitude:

Celebrations/Concerns:

Opportunities:

"The most terrifying thing is to accept oneself completely."

- C.G. Jung

Healing Habits:

Water   Movement
Meditation   Sleep
Clean Eating   Visualize
Oral Health   Quiet Alone

My Mantra:

Today's Intention: Date:

If I accepted my self completely, what would my day
look like?

Celebrations/Concerns: Gratitude:

Opportunities:

"And no one will listen to us until we listen to ourselves."
- Marianne Williamson

My Mantra: Healing Habits:

Water   Movement
Meditation   Sleep
Clean Eating   Visualize
Oral Health   Quiet Alone

Date _____

The best way to take care of myself today
is . . . .

Gratitude:

Celebrations/Concerns:

Opportunities:

'I am confident that nobody will accuse me of
selfishness if i ask to spend time, while i am still in good
health, with my family, my friends and also with
myself.'

       - Nelson Mandela

Healing Habits:

Water	Movement
Meditation	Sleep
Clean Eating	Visualize
Oral Health	Quiet Alone

My Mantra

Today's Intention: Date:

I am grateful for my relationship with . . .

Celebrations/Concerns: Gratitude:

Opportunities:

"One of the greatest regrets in life is being what others
would want you to be, rather than being yourself."
                                              - Shannon L. Alder

My Mantra: Healing Habits:

                                          Water   Movement
                                          Meditation   Sleep
                                          Clean Eating   Visualize
                                          Oral Health   Quiet Alone

Date:

What is one curiosity I can explore today?

Gratitude:

Celebrations/Concerns:

Opportunities:

"Beware of those who seek constant crowds, they are nothing alone."

— Charles Bukowski

Healing Habits:

Water   Movement
Meditation   Sleep
Clean Eating   Visualize
Oral Health   Quiet Alone

My Mantra:

Today's Intention: Date:

What do I need to do to have a deeper more sustainable
level of self-love?

Celebrations/Concerns: Gratitude:

Opportunities:

"Health is the crown on the well person's head that only
the ill person can see."

– Robin Sharma

My Mantra: Healing Habits:
                                               Water   Movement
                                               Meditation   Sleep
                                               Clean Eating   Visualize
                                               Oral Health   Quiet Alone

Date:

What is a personal challenge i can change?

Gratitude:

Celebrations/Concerns:

Opportunities:

"Self-compassion is key because when we're able to be gentle with ourselves in the midst of shame, we're more likely to reach out, connect, and experience empathy."

- Brene' Brown

Healing Habits:

Water   Movement
Meditation   Sleep
Clean Eating   Visualize
Oral Health   Quiet Alone

My Mantra:

Today's Intention: Date:

How can I be of service to others using compassion as
my guide?

Celebrations/Concerns: `   Gratitude:

Opportunities:

"How you love yourself is how you teach others to love
you"

- Rupi Kaur

My Mantra: Healing Habits:

Water   Movement
Meditation   Sleep
Clean Eating   Visualize
Oral Health   Quiet Alone

Date:

What tools do I need to acquire to feel more comfortable socially?

Gratitude:

Celebrations/Concerns:

Opportunities:

"It is not your job to like me - it's mine."
- Byron Katie

Healing Habits:

Water   Movement
Meditation   Sleep
Clean Eating   Visualize
Oral Health   Quiet Alone

My Mantra:

Today's Intention: Date:

With whom do I feel most at home?

Celebrations/Concerns: Gratitude:

Opportunities:

"I find there is a quality to being alone that is incredibly
precious. Life rushes back into the void, richer, more
vivid, fuller than before."
                              - Anne Morrow Lindbergh, Gift from the Sea

My Mantra: Healing Habits:
                                                    Water   Movement
                                                    Meditation   Sleep
                                                    Clean Eating   Visualize
                                                    Oral Health   Quiet Alone

Date:

What are the most important qualities of a positive and healthy friendship?

Gratitude:

Celebrations/Concerns:

Opportunities:

"If you learn to really sit with loneliness and embrace it for the gift that it is...an opportunity to get to know YOU, to learn how strong you really are, to depend on no one but YOU for your happiness...you will realize that a little loneliness goes a LONG way in creating a richer, deeper, more vibrant and colorful YOU."

· Mandy Hale

Healing Habits:

Water   Movement
Meditation   Sleep
Clean Eating   Visualize
Oral Health   Quiet Alone

My Mantra:

Today's Intention: Date:

What is one thing that I would change in my life if that
were possible?

Celebrations/Concerns: Gratitude:

Opportunities:

"Love yourself enough to live a healthy lifestyle."
- Jules Robson

My Mantra: Healing Habits:

Water	Movement
Meditation	Sleep
Clean Eating	Visualize
Oral Health	Quiet Alone

My ideal tribe would include people with these five qualities:

Gratitude:

Celebrations/Concerns:

Opportunities:

"To be nobody but yourself in a world which is doing its best, night and day, to make you everybody else means to fight the hardest battle which any human being can fight: and never stop fighting."
- E.E. Cummings

Healing Habits:

Water   Movement
Meditation   Sleep
Clean Eating   Visualize
Oral Health   Quiet Alone

My Mantra:

Today's Intention: Date:

Which is more important to be kind or to be right?

Celebrations/Concerns: Gratitude:

Opportunities:

"If a man does not keep pace with his companions,
perhaps it is because he hears a different drummer. Let
him keep steps to the music which he hears, however
measured or however far away."

- Henry David Thoreau

My Mantra: Healing Habits:

Water   Movement
Meditation   Sleep
Clean Eating   Visualize
Oral Health   Quiet Alone

Date:

What is something that I may need to rethink my position on?

Gratitude:

Celebrations/Concerns:

Opportunities:

"Don't worry if people think you're crazy. You are crazy. You have that kind of intoxicating insanity that lets other people dream outside of the lines and become who they're destined to be."
                                        - Jennifer Elisabeth

Healing Habits:

Water   Movement
Meditation   Sleep
Clean Eating   Visualize
Oral Health   Quiet Alone

My Mantra:

Today's Intention: Date:

What is the most surprising thing I've learned about
myself so far?

Celebrations/Concerns: Gratitude:

Opportunities:

"We are not held back by the love we didn't receive in the
past, but by the love we're not extending in the present."
                                        - Marianne Williamson

My Mantra: Healing Habits:
                                          Water   Movement
                                          Meditation   Sleep
                                          Clean Eating   Visualize
                                          Oral Health   Quiet Alone

Date

I am happiest when I . . . .

Gratitude:

Celebrations/Concerns:

Opportunities:

"Accept everything about yourself - I mean everything.
You are you and that is the beginning and the end - no
apologies, no regrets."

- Clark Moustakas

Healing Habits:

Water   Movement
Meditation   Sleep
Clean Eating   Visualize
Oral Health   Quiet Alone

My Mantra:

Today's Intention: Date

What is a signal i need to focus on self-care?

Celebrations/Concerns: Gratitude:

Opportunities:

"Your time is way too valuable to be wasting on people
that can't accept who you are."

- Turcois Ominek

My Mantra   Healing Habits:
                                          Water   Movement
                                          Meditation   Sleep
                                          Clean Eating   Visualize
                                          Oral Health   Quiet Alone

End of Month Check In

1. How do you feel physically? What needs attention? What has improved?

2. What is your level of self-compassion? What can you do to support deeper self-compassion? What is working right now? What needs focus?

3. What is your level of connection to yourself and others? Can you be of service to others in a positive manner? What is working? What needs focus?

Changing Habits

Old Habit

New Habit

New Action

Affirmation

pause

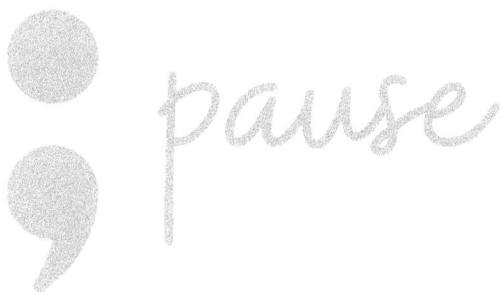

How do we graciously manage inevitable differences of opinion? Depending on the relationship, we sometimes have to find ways to work with others that challenge us. When we must get along, here are some ways to maintain our integrity:

pause

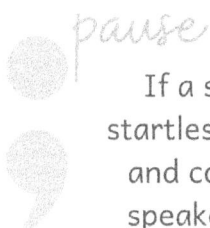

If a statement startles you, pause, and consider the speaker's intent.

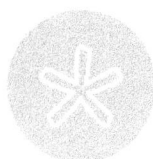

breathe

Take a breath. Step away you need to process.

Tell me more . . .

Allow the speaker to express their intent. If the speaker is sincere and respectful, ask for clarity.

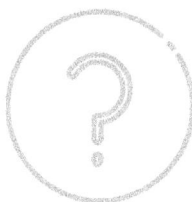

action

Gauge the speakers respect level. IF they are respectful, ask questions, if not, walk away.

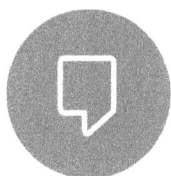

Press On

Use active listening skills to engage with respect. Equal speaking time is a good tool to use to determine mutual respect.

If you feel disrespected or you cannot be respectful, walk away.

change the subject

If the subject cannot be discussed with respect, change the subject.

walk away

Gratitude Invites Grace

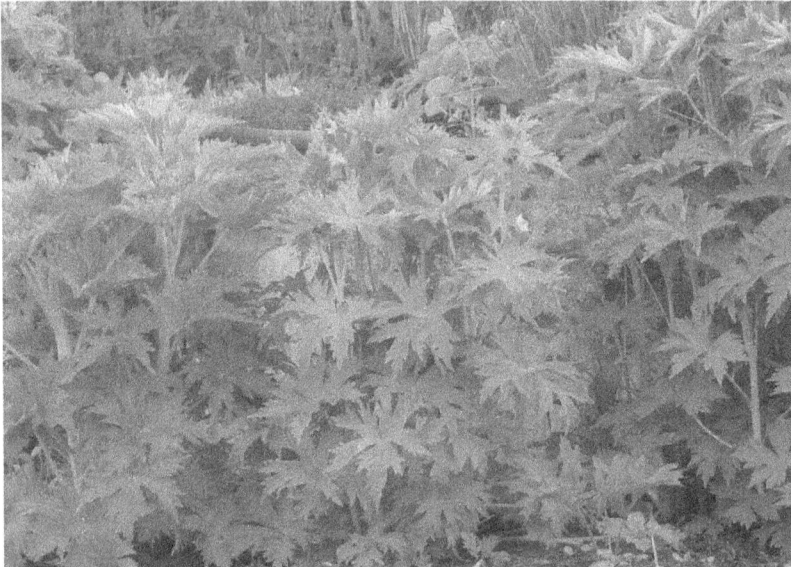

"Here's the gift of gratitude: In order to feel it, your ego has to take a backseat. What shows up in its place is greater compassion and understanding. Instead of being frustrated, you choose appreciation. And the more grateful you become, the more you have to be grateful for."

~ Oprah Winfrey

Book: *The Gifts OF Imperfection* by Brene' Brown

"Expressing gratitude has changed my life."

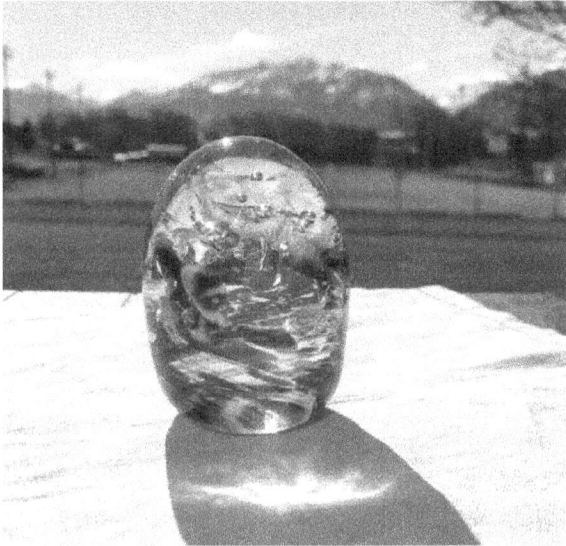

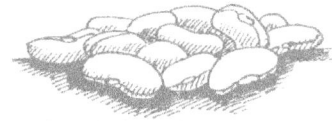

Find ways to create a habit of gratitude - Even on busy days - if you don't have time to journal - at least fill in 5 things you are grateful for - Throughout the day express gratitude to others!

An integral part of practicing gratitude is being aware of grace. Grace is when the universe provides what we neither expect nor deserve. It supersedes the law of cause and effect, where we do get what we deserve. Grace operates outside this ethical platform in response to gratitude. They operate in synergy, spinning off of one another with surprising results. We all have moments of grace when life seems to flow easily and without much effort, and other times when even tying a shoestring can be a challenge. We need to learn to get through life graciously whether we are "in-flow" or "out-of-flow," but wouldn't you choose to be in grace as much of the time as possible if you could? I would, and the path I use to get there is gratitude. Gratitude invites grace, and grace reinforces gratitude. I enjoy setting up opportunities for grace by practicing gratitude. It's the best way to start my day.

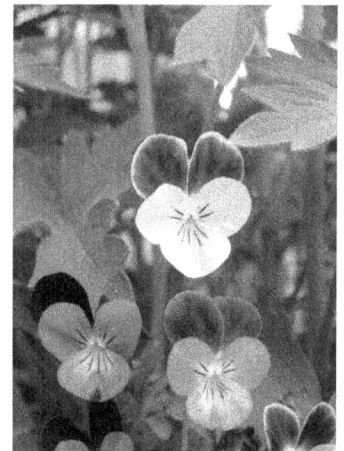

What makes your day flow best? A good night's sleep, clean, healthy eating, and healing habits are important, but expressing gratitude is an experiential way to live a grace-filled life.

Expressing gratitude has changed my life. If you do nothing else in your journal on busy days but fill in five things you are grateful for each day, I believe you will be supported in transforming your life. I wake up each morning and greet the day with gratitude before I even open my eyes. Often, I think of the things I'm so grateful for. In winter, it's that it's cool enough to be cozy and warm in lots of soft blankets. In summer, it's the delight of birds singing in the early summer morning before the sun even appears.

Gratitude has become a habit for me, just as eating healthy food clean, practicing good oral hygiene, and watering my garden are all habits. It is how I take care of my soul. Gratitude is an essential habit to develop, which is why it is incorporated into each page of your journal. This is an experiential journal, so I'd love for you to try the following for 30 days. Put 10 pennies into your right pocket. Throughout the day, whenever you think of something you are grateful for, transfer a penny to your left pocket. Give yourself 30 days of gratitude and see if your emotional responses to life as a result. Do you notice a shift in perspective?

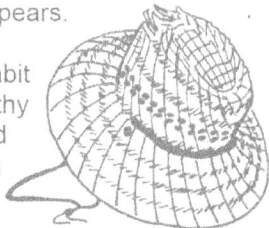

171

Who am I spiritually? How do I define spirituality?

Gratitude:

Celebrations/Concerns:

Opportunities:

"Gratitude unlocks the fullness of life. It turns what we have into enough and more. It turns denial into acceptance, chaos into order, and confusion into clarity. Gratitude makes sense of our past, brings peace for today, and creates a vision for tomorrow."
 - Melody Beattie

Healing Habits:

Water   Movement
Meditation   Sleep
Clean Eating   Visualize
Oral Health   Quiet Alone

My Mantra:

Today's Intention: Date:

What do I want to invite into my life?

Celebrations/Concerns: Gratitude:

Opportunities:

"Some people could be given an entire field of roses and only see the thorns in it. Others could be given a single weed and only see a wildflower in it. Perception is a key component to gratitude. And gratitude is the key to joy."
                                                — Amy Weatherly

My Mantra: Healing Habits:

                                          Water   Movement
                                          Meditation   Sleep
                                          Clean Eating   Visualize
                                          Oral Health   Quiet Alone

How can I be of service to others?

Gratitude:

Celebrations/Concerns:

Opportunities:

"We arrive at truth, not by reason only, but also by the heart."

- Blaise Pascal

Healing Habits:

Water   Movement
Meditation   Sleep
Clean Eating   Visualize
Oral Health   Quiet Alone

My Mantra:

Today's Intention: Date:

What am I most grateful for in my closest personal relationships?

Celebrations/Concerns: Gratitude:

Opportunities:

"There are cycles of success when things come to you and thrive, and cycles of failure, when they wither or disintegrate and you have to let them go in order to make room for new things to arise, or for transformation to happen"

- Eckhart Tolle

My Mantra: Healing Habits:

Water   Movement
Meditation   Sleep
Clean Eating Visualize
Oral Health Quiet Alone

What am i grateful for professionally?

Gratitude:

Celebrations/Concerns:

Opportunities:

"i want a singleness of eye, a purity of intention, a central core to my life that will enable me to carry out these obligations and activities as well as i can i want, in fact, to borrow from the language of the saints, to life 'in grace' as much of the time as possible"
- Anne Morrow Lindberg

Healing Habits:

Water   Movement
Meditation   Sleep
Clean Eating   Visualize
Oral Health   Quiet Alone

My Mantra:

Today's Intention: Date:

What childhood memory am I most grateful for?

Celebrations/Concerns: Gratitude:

Opportunities:

"And the day came when the risk to remain tight in a bud
was more painful than the risk it took to blossom."
                                              - Anais Nin

My Mantra: Healing Habits:

                                          Water   Movement
                                          Meditation   Sleep
                                          Clean Eating   Visualize
                                          Oral Health   Quiet Alone

What is my greatest strength physically?

Gratitude:

Celebrations/Concerns:

Opportunities:

"My religion is very simple. My religion is kindness."
- Dali Lama

Healing Habits:

Water   Movement
Meditation   Sleep
Clean Eating   Visualize
Oral Health   Quiet Alone

My Mantra:

Today's Intention: Date:

Am I able to view others with compassion rather than
judgment?

Celebrations/Concerns: Gratitude:

Opportunities:

"Keeping your body healthy is an expression of gratitude
to the whole cosmos - the trees, the clouds, everything."
                                    - Thich Nhat Hanh

My Mantra: Healing Habits:
                                      Water   Movement
                                      Meditation   Sleep
                                      Clean Eating   Visualize
                                      Oral Health   Quiet Alone

How can I express gratitude in my relationships?

Gratitude:

Celebrations/Concerns:

Opportunities:

"Beauty without grace is the hook without the bait"
- Ralph Waldo Emerson

Healing Habits:

Water   Movement
Meditation   Sleep
Clean Eating   Visualize
Oral Health   Quiet Alone

My Mantra:

Today's Intention: Date:

Write yourself a thank you letter, for an
unacknowledged accomplishment.

Celebrations/Concerns: Gratitude:

Opportunities:

"The really important thing is not to live, but to live well,
and to live well means the same thing as to live honorably
or rightly."

- Socrates

My Mantra: Healing Habits:

                                      Water   Movement
                                        Meditation   Sleep
                                        Clean Eating   Visualize
                                        Oral Health   Quiet Alone

What am I grateful for in nature?

Gratitude:

Celebrations/Concerns:

Opportunities:

"True forgiveness is when you can say, 'Thank you for that experience.'"

- Oprah Winfrey

Healing Habits:

Water
Meditation
Clean Eating
Oral Health

Movement
Sleep
Visualize
Quiet Alone

My Mantra:

Today's Intention: Date:

When I choose love, what can I accomplish today?

Celebrations/Concerns: Gratitude:

Opportunities:

"I am grateful for all those dark years, even though in retrospect they seem like a long bitter prayer that was answered finally."

– Marilynne Robinson

My Mantra: Healing Habits:

Water   Movement
Meditation   Sleep
Clean Eating   Visualize
Oral Health   Quiet Alone

Date

What am I most proud of in the last year?

Gratitude:

Celebrations/Concerns:

Opportunities:

"The ideal man bears the accidents of life with dignity and grace, making the best of circumstances."
                                    - Aristotle

Healing Habits:

Water   Movement
Meditation   Sleep
Clean Eating   Visualize
Oral Health   Quiet Alone

My Mantra:

Today's Intention: Date:

What skills do I have that I am most grateful for?

Celebrations/Concerns: Gratitude:

Opportunities:

"If you are not in control of your thoughts then you are
not in control of yourself."

- Thomas M. Sterner

My Mantra: Healing Habits:

Water   Movement
Meditation   Sleep
Clean Eating   Visualize
Oral Health   Quiet Alone

185

What physical comforts am i most grateful for?

Gratitude:

Celebrations/Concerns:

Opportunities:

"It can be a good thing, too, to learn to sit in your own weirdness."

- Sarah Wilson

Healing Habits:

Water   Movement
Meditation   Sleep
Clean Eating   Visualize
Oral Health   Quiet Alone

My Mantra:

Today's Intention: Date:

What is beautiful memory?

Celebrations/Concerns: Gratitude:

Opportunities:

"When you are spiritually connected, you are not looking
for occasions to be offended, and you are not judging
and labeling others. You are in a state of grace in which
you know you are connected to God and thus free
from the effects of anyone or anything external to
yourself."

                                                    - Wayne Dyer

My Mantra: Healing Habits:

                                        Water   Movement
                                        Meditation   Sleep
                                        Clean Eating   Visualize
                                        Oral Health   Quiet Alone

What abilities do I have that I am most grateful for?

Gratitude:

Celebrations/Concerns:

Opportunities:

"Gratitude makes sense of our past, brings peace for today, and creates a vision for tomorrow"
- Melody Beattie

Healing Habits:

Water   Movement
Meditation   Sleep
Clean Eating   Visualize
Oral Health   Quiet Alone

My Mantra:

Today's Intention: Date:

What gift was I given in childhood that I am most
grateful for?

Celebrations/Concerns: Gratitude:

Opportunities:

"Gratitude can transform common days into
thanksgivings, turn routine jobs into joy, and change
ordinary opportunities into blessings."
                                          - William Arthur Ward

My Mantra: Healing Habits:
                                        Water   Movement
                                        Meditation   Sleep
                                        Clean Eating   Visualize
                                        Oral Health   Quiet Alone

What skills would I be grateful to acquire?

Gratitude:

Celebrations/Concerns:

Opportunities:

"Give yourself a gift of five minutes of contemplation in awe of everything you see around you. Go outside and turn your attention to the many miracles around you. This five-minute-a-day regimen of appreciation and gratitude will help you to focus your life in awe."

- Wayne Dyer

Healing Habits:

Water   Movement
Meditation   Sleep
Clean Eating Visualize
Oral Health Quiet Alone

My Mantra:

Today's Intention: Date:

I call my Higher Power . . .

Celebrations/Concerns: Gratitude:

Opportunities:

"When grace is joined with wrinkles, it is adorable. There is an unspeakable dawn in happy old age."

— Victor Hugo

My Mantra: Healing Habits:

Water   Movement
Meditation   Sleep
Clean Eating   Visualize
Oral Health   Quiet Alone

How do I accept service from others?

Gratitude:

Celebrations/Concerns:

Opportunities:

"Act as if what you do makes a difference it does."
~ William James

Healing Habits:

Water   Movement
Meditation   Sleep
Clean Eating   Visualize
Oral Health   Quiet Alone

My Mantra:

Today's Intention: Date:

What self-care tools do I use daily that I am grateful
to have?

Celebrations/Concerns: Gratitude:

Opportunities:

"Gratitude is the healthiest of all human emotions. The
more you express gratitude for what you have, the
more likely you will have even more to express gratitude
for."

                                              - Zig Ziglar

My Mantra: Healing Habits:
                                        Water   Movement
                                        Meditation   Sleep
                                        Clean Eating   Visualize
                                        Oral Health   Quiet Alone

How does expressing gratitude often support stronger relationships?

Gratitude:

Celebrations/Concerns:

Opportunities:

"Most of the time one is discouraged by the work, but now and again by some grace something stands out and invites you to work on it, to elaborate it or animate it in some way. It's a mysterious process."

- Leonard Cohen

Water   Movement
Meditation   Sleep
Clean Eating   Visualize
Oral Health   Quiet Alone

Today's Intention: Date:

How can I show grace to another today?

Celebrations/Concerns: Gratitude:

Opportunities:

"It is through gratitude for the present moment that the
spiritual dimension of life opens up"

- Eckhart Tolle

My Mantra: Healing Habits:

Water   Movement
Meditation   Sleep
Clean Eating   Visualize
Oral Health   Quiet Alone

Is there something that I wish I had handled
with more grace in the past?

Gratitude:

Celebrations/Concerns:

Opportunities.

"At times our own light goes out and is rekindled by a
spark from another person. Each of us has cause to
think with deep gratitude of those who have lighted the
flame within us."

– Albert Schweitzer!

Healing Habits:

Water   Movement
Meditation   Sleep
Clean Eating   Visualize
Oral Health   Quiet Alone

My Mantra.

Today's Intention: Date:

If I had the chance for a 'do-over', what would it be?

Celebrations/Concerns: Gratitude:

Opportunities:

"Being a critic is easy. But if the critic tries to run the
operation, he soon understands that nothing is as easy as
his criticisms.
Criticism without a solution is merely an inflation of the
critic's ego"

- Haemin Sunim

My Mantra: Healing Habits:

Water   Movement
Meditation   Sleep
Clean Eating   Visualize
Oral Health   Quiet Alone

Three signs that I am living my best life
are . . .

Gratitude:

Celebrations/Concerns:

Opportunities:

"Denial helps us to pace our feelings of grief. There is
a grace in denial. It is nature's way of letting in only as
much as we can handle."

— Elisabeth Kubler-Ross

Water   Movement
Meditation   Sleep
Clean Eating Visualize
Oral Health Quiet Alone

Today's Intention: Date:

What is something I can learn about myself when someone's behavior triggers me?

Celebrations/Concerns: Gratitude:

Opportunities:

"For me, every hour is grace. And I feel gratitude in my heart each time I can meet someone and look at his or her smile."

- Elie Wiesel

My Mantra: Healing Habits:

Water   Movement
Meditation   Sleep
Clean Eating   Visualize
Oral Health   Quiet Alone

Define unconditional grace.

Gratitude:

Celebrations/Concerns:

Opportunities:

"Feeling gratitude and not expressing it is like wrapping a present and not giving it."

– William Arthur Ward

Healing Habits:

Water   Movement
Meditation   Sleep
Clean Eating Visualize
Oral Health Quiet Alone

My Mantra:

Date:

I model gratitude and grace is returned to me.

Celebrations/Concerns: Gratitude:

Opportunities:

"The amazing thing about love and attention and
encouragement and grace and success and joy is that
these things are infinite. We get a new supply every
single morning, and so we can give it away all day. We
never, ever have to monitor the supply of others or
grab or hoard"

                                        - Glennon Doyle Melton

My Mantra: Healing Habits:

                                        Water   Movement
                                        Meditation   Sleep
                                        Clean Eating   Visualize
                                        Oral Health   Quiet Alone

I am able to access compassion best
when . . . .

Gratitude:

Celebrations/Concerns:

Opportunities:

"Gratitude bestows reverence, allowing us to encounter
everyday epiphanies, those transcendent moments of
awe that change forever how we experience life and
the world."

- John Milton

Healing Habits:

Water	Movement
Meditation	Sleep
Clean Eating	Visualize
Oral Health	Quiet Alone

My Mantra:

End of Month Check In

1. How do you feel physically? What needs attention? What has improved?

2. What is your level of self-compassion? What can you do to support deeper self-compassion? What is working right now? What needs focus?

3. What is your level of connection to yourself and others? Can you be of service to others in a positive manner? What is working? What needs focus?

Changing Habits

Old Habit

New Habit

New Action

Affirmation

INVITING GRACE

Daily Practices
Journal gratitude daily.
Express gratitude to
others.

Gratitude Habit Builder:

Make gratitude a habit!

DEFINITIONS OF GRACE

- An Expression of Love.
- Beauty and Elegance in Movement
- Inner Dignity
- Ease of Flow in Life

MANIFESTING GRACE

- Offering Gratitude Daily
- Accepting Unconditional Love
- Open Mind & Heart
- Awareness of the
- Gifts of Nature
-

RECOGNIZING GRACE

- Recognition of Self in all beings
- Living Sincerely and Humbly
- Acts of Service
- Being Comfortable with Uncertainty

SIGNS OF GRACE MANIFESTED

- Unconditional Love
- Trusting Inner Wisdom
- Courage to be Disliked
- Forgiveness as Self-Care
- Inner Sense of Peace
- Everything you need is within!

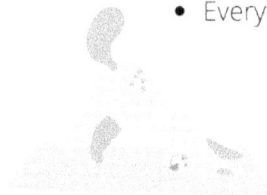

Courage, Grit, Curiosity

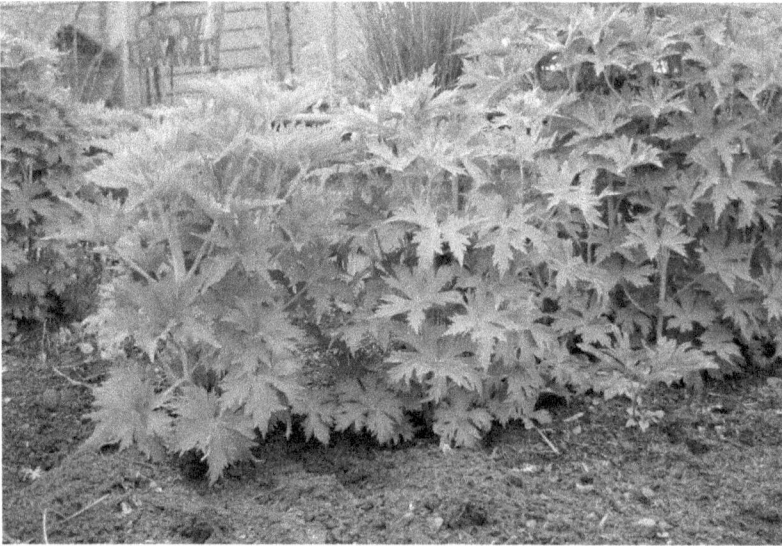

"What families have in common the world around is that they are the place where people learn who they are and how to be that way."

~ Jean Illsey Clarke

Book: *Untamed* by Glennon Doyal

"In times of uncertainty and in my best moments.."

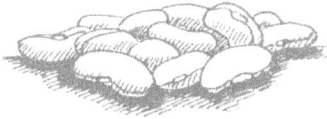

Fear manifests physically in all of us. Some of us grind our teeth when we are under extreme stress. When I was diagnosed in May of 2019, I broke 3 teeth in the first couple of months after the diagnosis. Dental guards are essential for me in times of deep stress.

In times of uncertainty and in my best moments, I approach life with courage, especially when faced with the unknown. However, I also love knowing what to expect, what is expected of me, and what is going to happen next. Yet, when confronted with uncertainty, I often try to morph it into its positive cousin, curiosity, which is another tool I love to use when I don't know what will happen next. I've been through enough trauma to know that there is always a silver lining somewhere in even the scariest times.

I know that I've gotten through bad times before, not always a shining beacon on a hill, but I'm still here, tarnished and bruised by the process. I've learned a few things about gut-wrenching fear yet doing the required anyway.

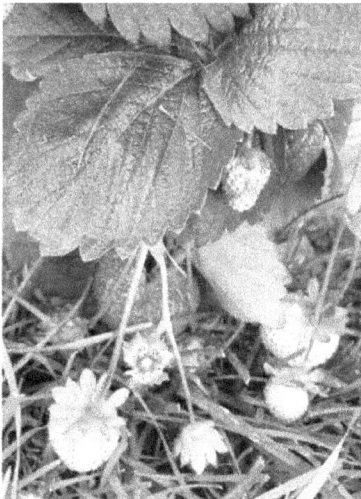

What I know for sure is that because of careful thought and planning, a fervent determination to heal, and the unfailing support of those who love me, I have made it through 100 % of the tough times.

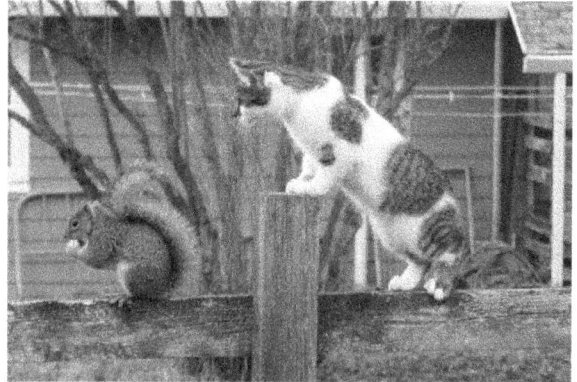

To achieve this outcome, however, I have had to give myself internal space to develop, to make the wrong choices and eventually stumble upon the right ones. We all need to face challenging situations on our own terms and reap the benefits based on our choices. It is common to want all the answers right now, but, often there simply are no answers, and you may not even know the right questions! But given time, the questions and their answers will arise and be settled. You can be done with this chapter, but you are not at the end of your story yet.

Life gives us so many opportunities to learn its lessons, to confront and conquer uncertainty. Journaling records our missteps and our victories. In journaling, we launch our ideas, only to have them boomerang back as consequences, sometimes favorable, sometimes not so favorable. Journaling also allows creatively problem-solving, the chance to try out different scenarios, and find the best outcomes. As we write our way to uncover our personal truths, we reinforce our own integrity, becoming the people that the universe had in mind. So, journaling is one way to build courage by exploring alternatives and tracking their consequences.

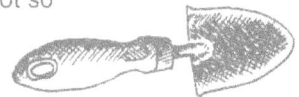

My hope for you is that you have created a morning ritual that includes journaling, deep breathing, moving your body, and the discovery of the amazing person that lies within.

Who am I in terms of courage and grit?

Gratitude:

Celebrations/Concerns:

Opportunities:

"It takes as much courage to have tried and failed as it does to have tried and succeeded"
- Anne Morrow Lindbergh

Healing Habits:

Water	Movement
Meditation	Sleep
Clean Eating	Visualize
Oral Health	Quiet Alone

My Mantra:

Today's Intention   Date:

What do I want for myself in terms of courage?

Celebrations/Concerns: Gratitude:

Opportunities:

                                          "Instead of fighting with your demons, examine them
                                          with curiosity and learn why they are there. Offer
                                          them love and understanding each and every time they
                                          come and visit."
                                                                              - Unknown

My Mantra   Healing Habits:
                                             Water   Movement
                                             Meditation   Sleep
                                             Clean Eating   Visualize
                                             Oral Health   Quiet Alone

How can I serve with courage?

Gratitude:

Celebrations/Concerns:

Opportunities:

"When I go into my garden with a spade and dig a bed, I feel such exhilaration and health that I discover that I have been defrauding myself all this time in letting others do for me what I should have done for myself."

- Emerson

Water   Movement
Meditation   Sleep
Clean Eating   Visualize
Oral Health   Quiet Alone

Today's Intention: Date:

I am curious about . . . .

Celebrations/Concerns: Gratitude:

Opportunities:

"As long as the sun smiles above us, our hopes will
always blossom."

- Atalay Aydin

My Mantra: Healing Habits:
                                           Water   Movement
                                           Meditation   Sleep
                                           Clean Eating   Visualize
                                           Oral Health   Quiet Alone

I demonstrate courage when i . . . .

Gratitude:

Celebrations/Concerns:

Opportunities:

"There are intersections of integrity and temptation in every career and every life. The challenge is to do the right thing no matter what."

— Bill Gates Sr.

Healing Habits

Water   Movement
Meditation   Sleep
Clean Eating   Visualize
Oral Health   Quiet Alone

My Mantra

Today's Intention: Date:

One of the most courageous things i have done in life is . . .

Celebrations/Concerns: Gratitude:

Opportunities:

"Courage does not always roar. Sometimes it's the quiet
voice saying, 'I will try again tomorrow.'"
                                   - Mary Anne Radmacher

My Mantra: Healing Habits:
                                        Water   Movement
                                        Meditation   Sleep
                                        Clean Eating Visualize
                                        Oral Health   Quiet Alone

Today's Intention

I wish I had the courage to . . . . .

Gratitude:

Celebrations/Concerns:

Opportunities:

"It takes courage to endure the sharp pains of self discovery rather than choose to take the dull pain of unconsciousness that would last the rest of our lives."
- Marianne Williamson

Healing Habits

Water   Movement
Meditation   Sleep
Clean Eating   Visualize
Oral Health   Quiet Alone

My Mantra

Date:

I am tenacious when it comes to . . . .

Celebrations/Concerns:

Gratitude:

Opportunities:

"Go confidently in the direction of your dreams! Live the life you've imagined - As you simplify your life, the laws of the universe will be simple."

- Henry David Thoreau

My Mantra

Healing Habits:

Water	Movement
Meditation	Sleep
Clean Eating	Visualize
Oral Health	Quiet Alone

I show curiosity towards fear when . . .

Gratitude:

Celebrations/Concerns:

Opportunities:

"Grit is choosing to lean in and work on your art
when the world thinks it's already good enough."
- Rob Beaudreault

Healing Habits:

Water   Movement
Meditation   Sleep
Clean Eating   Visualize
Oral Health   Quiet Alone

My Mantra:

Today's Intention: Date:

In times of uncertainty, what emotions do I experience
most?

Celebrations/Concerns: Gratitude:

Opportunities:

"Creative work is play. It is free speculation using the
materials of one's chosen form."

- Stephen Nachmanovitch

My Mantra: Healing Habits:

Water   Movement
Meditation   Sleep
Clean Eating   Visualize
Oral Health   Quiet Alone

217

i value courage most when . . .

Gratitude:

Celebrations/Concerns:

Opportunities:

"Our greatest happiness does not depend on the condition of life in which chance has placed us, but is always the result of a good conscience, good health, occupation, and freedom in all just pursuits."
- Thomas Jefferson

Healing Habits

Water	Movement
Meditation	Sleep
Clean Eating	Visualize
Oral Health	Quiet Alone

My Mantra:

Today's Intention:

Date:

I appreciate quiet moments alone because . . .

Celebrations/Concerns:

Gratitude:

Opportunities:

"Let me tell you this, if you meet a loner, no matter
what they tell you, it's not because they enjoy solitude.
It's because they have tried to blend into the world
before, and people continue to disappoint them"
- Jodi Picoult

My Mantra:

Healing Habits:
Water   Movement
Meditation   Sleep
Clean Eating   Visualize
Oral Health   Quiet Alone

If I knew I could not fail, what would I attempt?

Gratitude:

Celebrations/Concerns:

Opportunities:

"Grit is the grain of character. It may generally be described as heroism materialized, spirit and will thrust into heart, brain, and backbone, so as to form part of the physical substance of the man."
                                    - Edwin Percy Whipple

Healing Habits:

Water	Movement
Meditation	Sleep
Clean Eating	Visualize
Oral Health	Quiet Alone

My Mantra:

Today's Intention:

Date:

I would love to learn to . . . .

Celebrations/Concerns:

Gratitude:

Opportunities:

We waste so much energy trying to cover up who we are, when beneath every attitude is the want to be loved, and beneath every anger is a wound to be healed, and beneath every sadness is the fear that there will not be enough time."

- Mark Nepo

My Mantra:

Healing Habits:

Water   Movement
Meditation   Sleep
Clean Eating   Visualize
Oral Health   Quiet Alone

I demonstrate courage in my relationships
by . . . .

Gratitude:

Celebrations/Concerns:

Opportunities:

"Him that I love, I wish to be free -- even from me."
- Anne Morrow Lindbergh

Water
Meditation
Clean Eating
Oral Health

Movement
Sleep
Visualize
Quiet Alone

Today's Intention: Date:

I model courage when I . . . .

Celebrations/Concerns: Gratitude:

Opportunities:

"Over time, grit is what separates fruitful lives from aimlessness."

- John Ortberg

My Mantra: Healing Habits:

Water	Movement
Meditation	Sleep
Clean Eating	Visualize
Oral Health	Quiet Alone

My top 10 curiosities are:

Gratitude:

Celebrations/Concerns:

Opportunities:

"One does not become enlightened by imagining figures of light, but by making the darkness conscious. The latter procedure, however, is disagreeable and, therefore, not popular."

— C.G. Jung

Healing Habits:

Water   Movement
Meditation   Sleep
Clean Eating   Visualize
Oral Health   Quiet Alone

My Mantra:

Date:

Curiosity gives us space to explore. what are you curious about?

Celebrations/Concerns:

Gratitude:

Opportunities:

"It's amazing what we can do when our passion meet a purpose greater than ourself. That's why we need to explore our curiosity. Invest in what interests us. follow what intrigues us."

- Jay Shetty

My Mantra:

Healing Habits:

Water   Movement
Meditation   Sleep
Clean Eating   Visualize
Oral Health   Quiet Alone

Learning new things can feel ungraceful, I
am comfortable exploring my abilities.

Gratitude:

Celebrations/Concerns:

Opportunities:

"Life is a dance. Mindfulness is witnessing that dance."
- Amit Ray

Healing Habits

Water   Movement
Meditation   Sleep
Clean Eating   Visualize
Oral Health   Quiet Alone

My Mantra

Today's Intention: Date:

i choose to open my world to include things that take
hard work.

Celebrations/Concerns: Gratitude:

Opportunities:

"Grit is the persistence in following your own destiny."
- Paul Bradley Smith

My Mantra   Healing Habits

                                          Water   Movement
                                          Meditation   Sleep
                                          Clean Eating   Visualize
                                          Oral Health   Quiet Alone

Which friendships enrich my life?

Gratitude:

Celebrations/Concerns:

Opportunities:

'There are a thousand thousand reasons to live this life, everyone of them sufficient'
- Marilynne Robinson

Water   Movement
Meditation   Sleep
Clean Eating   Visualize
Oral Health   Quiet Alone

Today's Intention: Date:

I know I'm living my best life when I . . . .

Celebrations/Concerns: Gratitude:

Opportunities:

"In this moment, there is plenty of time. In this moment,
you are precisely as you should be. In this moment,
there is infinite possibility."

                                                    - Victoria Moran

My Mantra   Healing Habits:
                                                Water   Movement
                                                Meditation   Sleep
                                                Clean Eating   Visualize
                                                Oral Health   Quiet Alone

I show courage when I . . . . .

Gratitude:

Celebrations/Concerns:

Opportunities:

"Grit is knowing who you are and where you are headed, moving determinedly forward with eyes fixed on the mark, rather than the obstacles that lie in wait."
- Christine Bisch

Healing Habits:

Water	Movement
Meditation	Sleep
Clean Eating	Visualize
Oral Health	Quiet Alone

My Mantra

It took courage to choose . . .

Celebrations/Concerns: Gratitude:

Opportunities:

"You gain strength, courage, and confidence by every
experience in which you really stop to look fear in the
face. You are able to say to yourself, 'I lived through
this horror. I can take the next thing that comes along."
                                              - Eleanor Roosevelt

My Mantra:

Healing Habits:
  Water   Movement
  Meditation   Sleep
  Clean Eating   Visualize
  Oral Health   Quiet Alone

I have gotten through tough times before.
One tool I use is . . . .

Gratitude:

Celebrations/Concerns:

Opportunities:

"The human capacity for burden is like bamboo - far
more flexible than you'd ever believe at first glance."
- Jodi Picoult

Healing Habits:

Water	Movement
Meditation	Sleep
Clean Eating	Visualize
Oral Health	Quiet Alone

My Mantra:

Today's Intention: Date:

I can say no to _____ because . . . . .

Celebrations/Concerns: Gratitude:

Opportunities:

"The oak fought the wind and was broken, the willow
bent when it must and survived."

- Robert Jordan

My Mantra   Healing Habits:

                                  Water   Movement
                                  Meditation   Sleep
                                  Clean Eating   Visualize
                                  Oral Health   Quiet Alone

I can always count on . . . .

Gratitude:

Celebrations/Concerns:

Opportunities:

"Life is messy. Grit and grace come at us fast, side by side. Sometimes the grit becomes overwhelming and diminishes our spirit. What's good seems lost and gone forever. This is a story about the pathway back to what's beautiful when the way back seems impossible."
- Sharon E. Rainey

Healing Habits:

Water	Movement
Meditation	Sleep
Clean Eating	Visualize
Oral Health	Quiet Alone

My Mantra

Today's Intention: Date:

What time of day is my courage level the highest?

Celebrations/Concerns: Gratitude:

Opportunities:

"Thank you flower... For showing me how to grow even
while being blocked from the sun by the tall redwoods,
having to find ways around and through, so my sunshine
heart could glow into me, becoming the blossom that is
watered and needed, and listened to, and sung to sleep
in peaceful loving arms. Thank you for awakening me
to my life."

                                              - Bodhi Smith

My Mantra: Healing Habits:
                                       Water   Movement
                                       Meditation   Sleep
                                       Clean Eating   Visualize
                                       Oral Health   Quiet Alone

if I don't have courage at the moment, I can pause. Today I will pause if I need to.

Gratitude:

Celebrations/Concerns:

Opportunities:

"Persistence and resilience only come from having been given the chance to work through difficult problems."

- Gever Tulley

Healing Habits:

Water	Movement
Meditation	Sleep
Clean Eating	Visualize
Oral Health	Quiet Alone

My Mantra:

Date:

I can use curiosity to see new possibilities. Today I will explore . .

Celebrations/Concerns:

Gratitude:

Opportunities:

"Men are developed the same way gold is mined. When gold is mined, several tons of dirt must be moved to get an ounce of gold, but one doesn't go into the mine looking for dirt-one goes in looking for the gold."
- Andrew Carnegie

My Mantra:

Healing Habits:

Water	Movement
Meditation	Sleep
Clean Eating	Visualize
Oral Health	Quiet Alone

End of Month Check In

1. How do you feel physically? What needs attention? What has improved?

2. What is your level of self-compassion? What can you do to support deeper self-compassion? What is working right now? What needs focus?

3. What is your level of connection to yourself and others? Can you be of service to others in a positive manner? What is working? What needs focus?

Changing Habits

Old Habit

New Habit

New Action

Affirmation

COURAGEOUS CONVERSATIONS
COMMUNICATING WITH CURIOSITY

| WHO ? | WHAT? |
| WHERE? | WHEN? |

Clearly Identify the Problem

- Have you tried to look at this issue from multiple points of view?
- What has been said?
- Did you interpret the *intention* of the speaker correctly?
- Have you asked for clarification?

- Is this issue worth addressing?
- What is the best case scenario for this conversation?
- What is the worst case scenario?
- Know *why* you want to have this conversation.

- When is the best time and place for this conversation?
- How important is this person to you personally or professionally?
- What is your primary motivation to have this conversation?
- Will this conversation help or hurt my relationship?

Outcome:
- Did this conversation go the way I had hoped?
- Was I able to be clear, concise and honest in my communication?
- What would I do differently next time?

Heal Your Body

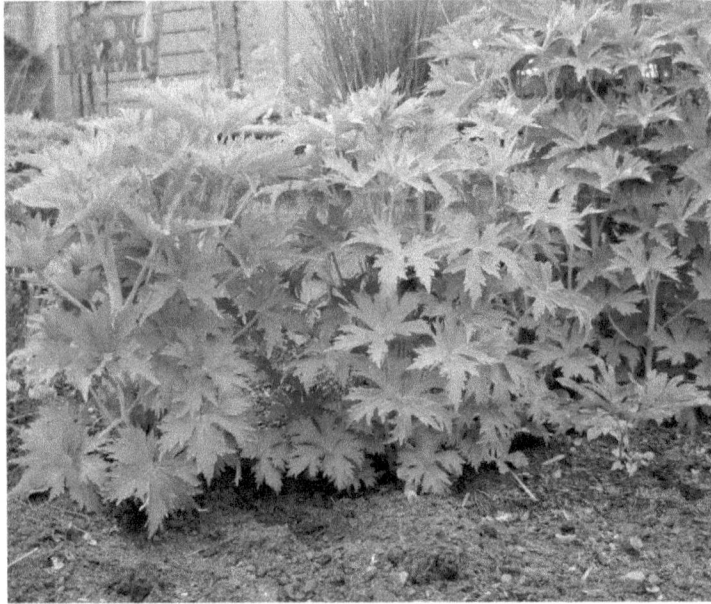

""Our most natural state is joy. It is the foundation for love, compassion, healing, and the desire to alleviate suffering."

~Deepak Chopra

Book: *The Healing Self* by Deepak Chopra M.D. & Rudolph E. Tanzi PhD

"I was reeling with fear and confusion.."

My walk through medical complexities has never been easy, though I am beginning to find my way through it. After multiple life-threatening diagnoses, I have emerged from several near-death encounters. Figuring out what really ailed me was the biggest problem of all, with countless distractions keeping me from that essential discovery. In the aftermath, I see now that it was allowing self-love to guide my recovery, using meditation, diet, and journaling to inform my recovery. Today, I use meditation and journaling as my inward excavator and a practical arrangement with food to safeguard my health. If food does not heal, it is not part of my diet, it's as simple as that. I choose to eat and drink what heals, not hurts my body.

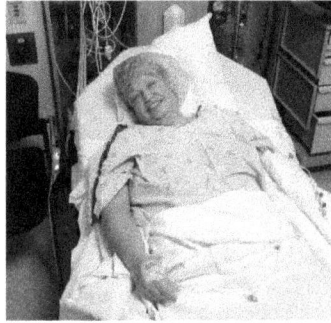

However, what works for me might not work for you. Bio-Individuality is an important concept to consider when discovering how your body works best. Tracking your own body's responses to various food types can help isolate what works best for you. One of the best ways to determine this is by tracking your food responses through journaling. You may see drastic weight regulation, blood sugar improvement, less joint pain, and a host of other physical advantages by eating the right food for your body. Your body is your best ally for lifestyle changes. Its feedback is spot on. Strangely enough, whenever I eat a really healthy salad with all the fresh fruits and veggies that my body loves, I actually feel my body purr like a well-satiated cat. Much of what I eat comes straight from my own garden. Over time, Tom and I have converted our somewhat confined back yard into a nutritional field of delights, which has become the source of our year-round diet. Our garden is packed with nutritional food that makes up the majority of our meals. Their seasonal freshness simply can't be beat.

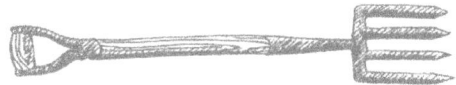

I would encourage you to use meditation and journaling to discover your personal nutritional gold mines and begin stroking the purring cat within. Start listing the foods that you eat every day and ranking their efficiency against your body's response to them. How healthy do you feel after you eat them? How long-lasting is a positive result? What other forms of this food might your body respond well to?

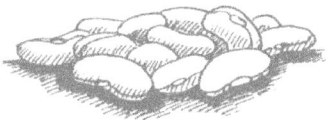

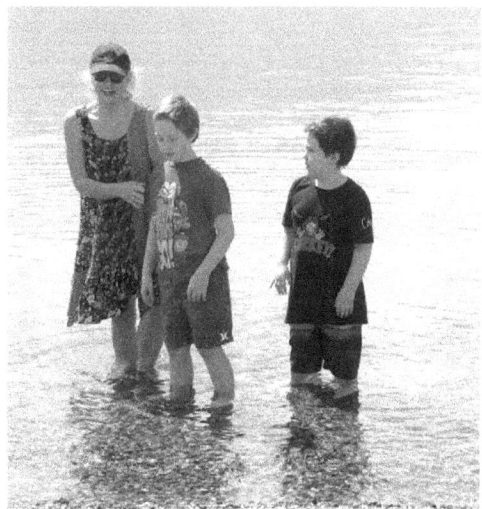

Organic is expensive and most of us need to be careful about spending. If you can not afford to be completely organic in your household, check out the Dirty Dozen and the Clean 15, it is updated yearly to keep you up to date on safe farming practices. Visit Greenmatters.com

241

Who am I physically?

Gratitude:

Celebrations/Concerns:

Opportunities:

"Your health is what you make of it. Everything you do and think either adds to the vitality, energy and spirit you possess or takes away from it."

— Ann Wigmore

Healing Habits

Water   Movement
Meditation   Sleep
Clean Eating   Visualize
Oral Health   Quiet Alone

My Mantra:

Today's Intention: Date:

What do I want to heal in my body?

Celebrations/Concerns: Gratitude:

Opportunities:

"I know you think this world is too dark to even dream
in color, but I've seen flowers bloom at midnight. I've
seen kites fly in gray skies and they were real close
to looking like the sunrise, and sometimes it takes the
most wounded wings, the most broken things to notice
how strong the breeze it, how precious the flight."
                                              - Andrea Gibson

My Mantra   Healing Habits:
                                      Water   Movement
                                      Meditation   Sleep
                                      Clean Eating   Visualize
                                      Oral Health   Quiet Alone

How can I best serve in spite of any
physical limitations i might have?

Gratitude:

Celebrations/Concerns:

Opportunities:

"The scientific truth may be put quite briefly, eat
moderately, having an ordinary mixed diet, and don't
worry."

- Robert Hutchison

Healing Habits:

Water   Movement
Meditation   Sleep
Clean Eating   Visualize
Oral Health   Quiet Alone

My Mantra:

Today's Intention: Date:

What habit best benefits my health?

Celebrations/Concerns: Gratitude:

Opportunities:

"Happiness is nothing more than good health and a bad memory."

- Albert Schweitzer

My Mantra: Healing Habits:

                                                      Water   Movement
                                                      Meditation   Sleep
                                                      Clean Eating   Visualize
                                                      Oral Health   Quiet Alone

245

What habit no longer serves me? What do I need to do to change it?

Gratitude:

Celebrations/Concerns:

Opportunities:

"Physical fitness is not only one of the most important keys to a healthy body, it is the basis of dynamic and creative intellectual activity."

– John F. Kennedy

Healing Habits:

Water   Movement
Meditation   Sleep
Clean Eating   Visualize
Oral Health   Quiet Alone

My Mantra:

Today's Intention: Date:

I believe what I put in my body can heal it or hurt it,
today I choose . . .

Celebrations/Concerns: Gratitude:

Opportunities:

"Healing takes courage, and we all have courage, even
if we have to dig a little to find it."

- Tori Amos

My Mantra: Healing Habits:

Water   Movement
Meditation   Sleep
Clean Eating   Visualize
Oral Health   Quiet Alone

Sleep restores my health, my sleep is . . . .

Gratitude:

Celebrations/Concerns:

Opportunities:

"By cleansing your body on a regular basis and eliminating toxins from your environment, your body can begin to heal itself, prevent disease, and become more strong and resilient than you ever thought possible."

- Dr. Sebi

Healing Habits:

Water
Meditation
Clean Eating
Oral Health

Movement
Sleep
Visualize
Quiet Alone

My Mantra:

Date:

When I have complete food freedom i will . . .

Celebrations/Concerns:

Gratitude:

Opportunities:

"Eat to live, not live to eat."
- Socrates

My Mantra:

Healing Habits:

Water   Movement
Meditation   Sleep
Clean Eating   Visualize
Oral Health   Quiet Alone

Date

What skill do I need to learn to support my healing most?

Gratitude:

Celebrations/Concerns:

Opportunities:

"Healing yourself is connected with healing others."
- Yoko Ono

Healing Habits:

Water   Movement
Meditation   Sleep
Clean Eating   Visualize
Oral Health   Quiet Alone

My Mantra:

Today's Intention: Date:

I can improve the quality of my life by adding more
..... in my life

Celebrations/Concerns: Gratitude:

Opportunities:

"Love is not as important as good health. You cannot be
in love if you're not healthy. You can't appreciate it."
                                        - Bryan Cranston

My Mantra: Healing Habits:
                                      Water   Movement
                                      Meditation   Sleep
                                      Clean Eating   Visualize
                                      Oral Health   Quiet Alone

When I see my reflection I feel . . . .

Gratitude:

Celebrations/Concerns:

Opportunities:

"The doctor of the future will give no medicines, but will interest his patients in the care of the human frame, in diet, and in the causes and prevention of disease."

- Thomas Edison

Healing Habits:

Water   Movement
Meditation   Sleep
Clean Eating   Visualize
Oral Health   Quiet Alone

My Mantra:

Today's Intention: Date:

My favorite healthy meal is

Celebrations/Concerns: Gratitude:

Opportunities:

"Healthy citizens are the greatest asset any country
can have."

- Winston Churchill

My Mantra: Healing Habits:

Water   Movement
Meditation   Sleep
Clean Eating   Visualize
Oral Health   Quiet Alone

I drink enough water to flush toxins from my body daily.

Gratitude:

Celebrations/Concerns:

Opportunities:

"I've experienced several different healing methodologies over the years - counseling, self-help seminars, and I've read a lot - but none of them will work unless you really want to heal."
— Lindsay Wagner

Healing Habits:

Water   Movement
Meditation   Sleep
Clean Eating   Visualize
Oral Health   Quiet Alone

My Mantra:

Today's Intention: Date:

Using fasting as a healing modality is something i . . .

Celebrations/Concerns: Gratitude:

Opportunities:

"Let your body be your holy temple."
- Lailah Gifty Akita

My Mantra: Healing Habits:
                                              Water   Movement
                                              Meditation   Sleep
                                              Clean Eating   Visualize
                                              Oral Health   Quiet Alone

I would love to learn . . . .

Gratitude:

Celebrations/Concerns:

Opportunities:

"Garbage in garbage out."
- George Fuechsel

Water   Movement
Meditation   Sleep
Clean Eating   Visualize
Oral Health   Quiet Alone

Today's Intention: Date:

I feel best when I eat

Celebrations/Concerns: Gratitude:

Opportunities:

"It has been said that time heals all wounds. The truth is
that time does not heal anything. It merely passes. It is
what we do during the passing of time that helps or
hinders the healing process."

- Jay Marshall

My Mantra: Healing Habits:

                                              Water   Movement
                                              Meditation   Sleep
                                              Clean Eating   Visualize
                                              Oral Health   Quiet Alone

Date:

My favorite self-care activity is . . . .

Gratitude:

Celebrations/Concerns:

Opportunities:

'if you think wellness is expensive, try illness'
- Unknown

Healing Habits:

Water   Movement
Meditation   Sleep
Clean Eating   Visualize
Oral Health   Quiet Alone

My Mantra:

Today's Intention: Date:

Sexual health is important to balance, my interest level
in sex is . . . .

Celebrations/Concerns: Gratitude:

Opportunities:

"Where you tend a rose, my lad, a thistle cannot grow."
                                    - Francess Hodgson Burnett

My Mantra: Healing Habits:
                                      Water   Movement
                                      Meditation   Sleep
                                      Clean Eating   Visualize
                                      Oral Health   Quiet Alone

Date:

My ultimate health dream is . . .

Gratitude:

Celebrations/Concerns:

Opportunities:

"There are some remedies worse than the disease."
- Publilius Syrus

Healing Habits:

Water   Movement
Meditation   Sleep
Clean Eating   Visualize
Oral Health   Quiet Alone

My Mantra:

Today's Intention: Date:

The last time i was the recipient of an unexpected
random act of kindness i

Celebrations/Concerns: Gratitude:

Opportunities:

"By far the strongest poison to the human spirit is the
inability to forgive oneself or another person.
Forgiveness is no longer an option but a necessity for
healing."

- Caroline Myss

My Mantra: Healing Habits:

                                            Water   Movement
                                            Meditation   Sleep
                                            Clean Eating Visualize
                                            Oral Health Quiet Alone

Date: _____

A perfect day for me would include . . . .

Gratitude:

Celebrations/Concerns:

Opportunities:

"Those who think they have no time for healthy eating
will sooner or later have to find time for illness."
- Edward Stanley

Healing Habits:

Water   Movement
Meditation   Sleep
Clean Eating Visualize
Oral Health Quiet Alone

My Mantra:

Today's Intention: Date:

If I could eliminate one health challenge it would
be . . .

Celebrations/Concerns: Gratitude:

Opportunities:

"When diet is wrong medicine is of no use
When diet is correct medicine is of no need"
- Ancient Ayurvedic Proverb

My Mantra: Healing Habits:
                                                Water   Movement
                                                Meditation   Sleep
                                                Clean Eating   Visualize
                                                Oral Health   Quiet Alone

Date:

My favorite way to move my body is . . . .

Gratitude:

Celebrations/Concerns:

Opportunities:

"The place of true healing is a fierce place. It's a giant place. It's a place of monstrous beauty and endless dark and glimmering light. And you have to work really, really, really hard to get there, but you can do it."
                                    - Cheryl Strayed

Healing Habits:

Water   Movement
Meditation   Sleep
Clean Eating   Visualize
Oral Health   Quiet Alone

My Mantra:

Today's Intention: Date:

I incorporate joy daily . . .

Celebrations/Concerns: Gratitude:

Opportunities:

"The food you eat can be either the safest and most
powerful form of medicine or the slowest form of
poison."

                                                        - Ann Wigmore

My Mantra: Healing Habits:

                                                   Water   Movement
                                                   Meditation   Sleep
                                                   Clean Eating   Visualize
                                                   Oral Health   Quiet Alone

Music heals, I listen to music to adjust my attitude.

Gratitude:

Celebrations/Concerns:

Opportunities:

"Sorry, there's no magic bullet. You gotta eat healthy and live healthy to be healthy and look healthy. End of story."

- Morgan Spurlock.

Healing Habits:

Water   Movement
Meditation   Sleep
Clean Eating   Visualize
Oral Health   Quiet Alone

My Mantra:

Today's Intention: Date:

My last fun adrenaline rush was . . .

Celebrations/Concerns   Gratitude:

Opportunities:

"Your diet is a bank account. Good food choices are
good investments."

- Bethenny Frankel

My Mantra   Healing Habits:

Water   Movement
Meditation   Sleep
Clean Eating   Visualize
Oral Health   Quiet Alone

My favorite body part is . . .

Gratitude:

Celebrations/Concerns:

Opportunities:

"Healing is an art. It takes time, it takes practice. It takes love."

- Maza Dohta

Healing Habits:

Water	Movement
Meditation	Sleep
Clean Eating	Visualize
Oral Health	Quiet Alone

My Mantra:

Today's Intention   Date:

It is a challenge to love my

Celebrations/Concerns: Gratitude:

Opportunities:

"Follow your inner moonlight."
~ Allen Ginsberg

My Mantra: Healing Habits:
                                                  Water   Movement
                                                  Meditation   Sleep
                                                  Clean Eating   Visualize
                                                  Oral Health   Quiet Alone

An activity that always brings me joy is . . .

Gratitude:

Celebrations/Concerns:

Opportunities:

"Don't allow a love problem or work problem to become an eating problem. Stop trying to stuff your feelings down with food."

– Karen Salmansohn

Water   Movement
Meditation   Sleep
Clean Eating   Visualize
Oral Health   Quiet Alone

Today's Intention: Date:

I can honor my sexuality in a healthy manner by . . .

Celebrations/Concerns: Gratitude:

Opportunities.

"Laughter is important, not only because it makes us
happy, it also has actual health benefits. And that's
because laughter completely engages the body and
releases the mind. It connects us to others, and that in
itself has a healing effect."

- Marlo Thomas

My Mantra.   Healing Habits:

                                              Water   Movement
                                              Meditation   Sleep
                                              Clean Eating   Visualize
                                              Oral Health   Quiet Alone

271

I feel most myself when I . . .

Gratitude:

Celebrations/Concerns:

Opportunities:

"If you are depressed you are living in the past. If you
are anxious you are living in the future. If you are at
peace you are living in the present."

— Sarah Wilson

Healing Habits:

Water	Movement
Meditation	Sleep
Clean Eating	Visualize
Oral Health	Quiet Alone

My Mantra:

End of Month Check In

1. How do you feel physically? What needs attention? What has improved?

2. What is your level of self-compassion? What can you do to support deeper self-compassion? What is working right now? What needs focus?

3. What is your level of connection to yourself and others? Can you be of service to others in a positive manner? What is working? What needs focus?

Changing Habits

Old Habit

New Habit

New Action

Affirmation

Elimination Diet: Food Tracker

Too often, our bodies react to food in unfavorable ways, either through allergies, sensitivities, or because of resident toxins. As you modify your diet, it's important to track your body's responses to these changes. Bodily reactivity could be physical, emotional, and behavioral. Each of us is sensitive to different things so you cannot easily follow a 'list' of inflammatory foods to avoid and discover how your body reacts. I'd like to suggest removing processed, sugar-filled foods and replacing them with more unrefined versions of the foods you enjoy. A simple rule of thumb: Go organic whenever possible.

Food Symptom Tracker

Skin Issues

Headache

Bloating / Gas

Joint Pain

Itchiness

Irritability

Flushing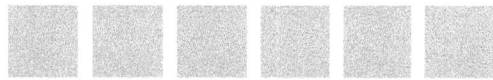

Restless Body

Attention Issues

Hair, Nail Issues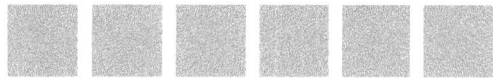

Wonder & Hope

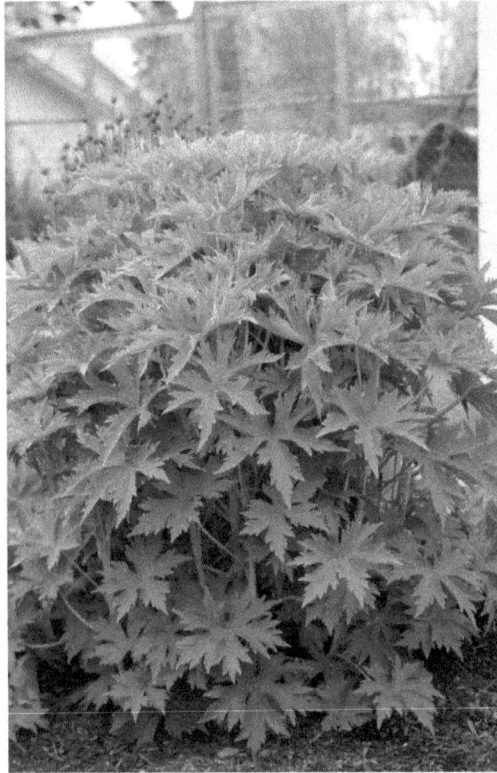

"There are two types of seeds in the mind: those that create anger, fear, frustration, jealousy, hatred and those that create love, compassion, equanimity and joy. Spirituality is germination and sprouting of the second group and transforming the first group."

~ Amit Ray

Book: *Wired for Healing* by Anne Hopper

"I use wonder to explore possibilities."

I use wonder to explore possibilities. It empowers the principle of non-attachment, which frees us from disappointment and the rigidity that comes when we latch onto only one solution to an obstacle. The freedom of leaving an outcome open to what develops is a gift when the alternative is trying to force your will, regardless of any others that may be affected by your desired outcome. Wonder gives us space and time to problem solve in a positive mindset. "I wonder if I'll get the job," or "Is there something that is a better fit?," as opposed to "If I don't get that job I'll just die!" Can you see the difference in the energy of both those statements? In many ways, being open to alternatives is more realistic in how we synchronize with the rhythms of the universe.

Wonderment is somewhat new to me, however. In the past I have allowed fear to overwhelm me, to freeze me, and to alter my life to avoid an unpleasant situation. By realizing and more deeply accepting how little control I actually have has imparted an inner peace that is not easily shaken. During this global crisis, this unconfining sense of wonder has been quite helpful. "I wonder if I'll be able to celebrate my 60th birthday with others, or if I should celebrate it in solitude this year?" or, "I wonder if my grandsons will return to school in the fall, or if I should start creating an interest-based curriculum for them now?" Rather than limiting options, wonder creates them.

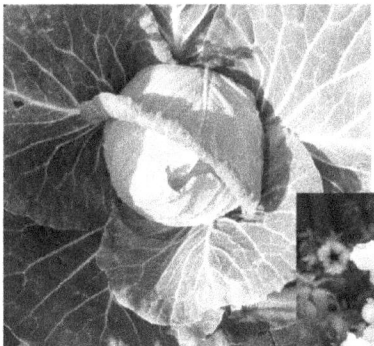

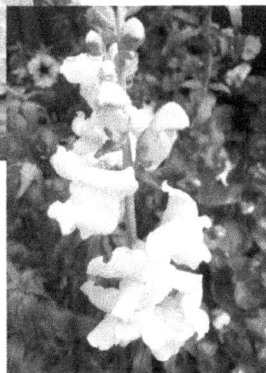

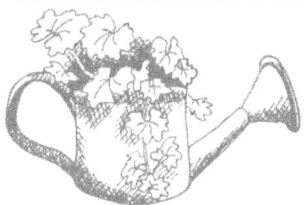

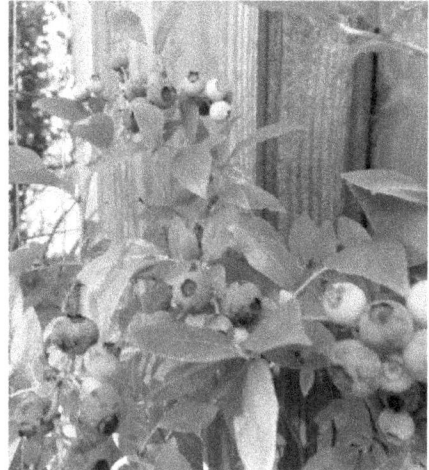

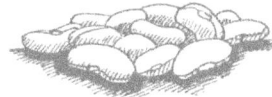

Neurotoxins are common in foods, and medications. Artificial colors, chemicals in processed foods, and artificial vitamins are just some of the issues in our ever-growing population of those with chronic mystery illnesses. Read the labels. Vote with your dollars. Resist bad food.

What is the role of wonder in your life? How can you shift your thinking to reduce the fear factors and remain clear-headed and open to possibilities? When you become an observer of your thoughts, it is much easier to consider other perspectives, other points of view that are better considered. By allowing ourselves to wonder, to extend our understanding of non-attachment to open-ended outcomes, we can drain the drama from situations and allow them to resolve more organically.

I'd like to suggest incorporating wonder into your next uncertain circumstance and see if it neutralizes the fear factor. Remember to choose love, the instrument for positive outcomes. And if it doesn't go the way you expect, you might want to get ready for a welcome surprise!

Date: _____

Who am I emotionally?

Gratitude:

Celebrations/Concerns:

Opportunities:

"Joy is what happens to us when we allow ourselves to
recognize how good things really are."
                                    - Marianne Williamson

Healing Habits:

Water   Movement
Meditation   Sleep
Clean Eating   Visualize
Oral Health   Quiet Alone

My Mantra:

Today's Intention: Date:

How do i want my best life to look?

Celebrations/Concerns: Gratitude:

Opportunities:

"Look up at the stars and not down at your feet. Try
to make sense of what you see, and wonder about
what makes the universe exist. Be curious"
                                              - Stephen Hawking

My Mantra: Healing Habits:
                                                Water   Movement
                                                Meditation   Sleep
                                                Clean Eating   Visualize
                                                Oral Health   Quiet Alone

Date: _____

How can I be of service?

Gratitude:

Celebrations/Concerns:

Opportunities:

"Laughter is the sun that drives the winter from the human face."

- Victor Hugo

Healing Habits:

Water   Movement
Meditation   Sleep
Clean Eating   Visualize
Oral Health   Quiet Alone

My Mantra:

Today's Intention: Date:

I choose to experience hope as a positive space in
which to explore possibilities. Today I hope for...

Celebrations/Concerns: Gratitude:

Opportunities:

"He who can no longer pause to wonder and stand rapt
in awe is as good as dead, his eyes are closed -
                                              - Albert Einstein

My Mantra: Healing Habits:
                                                  Water   Movement
                                                  Meditation   Sleep
                                                  Clean Eating   Visualize
                                                  Oral Health   Quiet Alone

Date:

I choose to remain unattached to the
outcome, I wonder what . . .

Gratitude:

Celebrations/Concerns:

Opportunities:

"It isn't that they can't see the solution, it is that they
can't see the problem."

- Gilbert K. Chesterton

Healing Habits:

Water   Movement
Meditation   Sleep
Clean Eating   Visualize
Oral Health   Quiet Alone

My Mantra:

Today's Intention: Date:

One dream I am exploring is

Celebrations/Concerns: Gratitude:

Opportunities:

Wisdom begins in wonder.
- Socrates

My Mantra: Healing Habits:
                                                  Water   Movement
                                                  Meditation   Sleep
                                                  Clean Eating   Visualize
                                                  Oral Health   Quiet Alone

What have i accomplished that did not seem possible a couple of months ago?

Gratitude:

Celebrations/Concerns:

Opportunities:

"Our most basic assumption is that we are the way we see ourselves and the world is the way we see it. We are taught to believe life SHOULD be a certain way and we SHOULD be a certain way. When it isn't and we aren't, we assume there's something wrong and something should be done to fix things. Suffering happens when we want life to be OTHER than the way it is."

- Cheri Huber

Healing Habits:

Water   Movement
Meditation   Sleep
Clean Eating   Visualize
Oral Health   Quiet Alone

My Mantra:

Today's Intention: Date:

What is one thing that makes me GLOW?

Celebrations/Concerns: Gratitude:

Opportunities:

"When we stop chasing the wind, we can begin to
live in peace."

- Wayne Muller

My Mantra: Healing Habits:
                                                  Water   Movement
                                                  Meditation   Sleep
                                                  Clean Eating   Visualize
                                                  Oral Health   Quiet Alone

How do I provide value to my community?

Gratitude:

Celebrations/Concerns:

Opportunities:

"Sometimes I wonder if we shall ever grow up in our politics and say definite things which mean something, or whether we shall always go on using generalities to which everyone can subscribe, and which mean very little."

- Eleanor Roosevelt

Healing Habits:

Water   Movement
Meditation   Sleep
Clean Eating   Visualize
Oral Health   Quiet Alone

My Mantra:

Today's Intention: Date:

What strength would I like to develop further?

Celebrations/Concerns: Gratitude:

Opportunities:

"Our world is in crisis because of our perception: how
we see the world creates the world in which we live.
Ultimately, it's about each one of us taking the
responsibility of being the Presence of God."

— Walter Starcke

My Mantra: Healing Habits:

Water   Movement
Meditation   Sleep
Clean Eating   Visualize
Oral Health   Quiet Alone

Date: Today's Intention

What is a small pleasure that I can experience daily?

Gratitude: Celebrations/Concerns:

Opportunities:

"There is nothing enlightened about shrinking so that other people won't feel insecure around you. We are all meant to shine, as children do."

- Marianne Williamson

Healing Habits: My Mantra:

Water   Movement

Meditation   Sleep

Clean Eating   Visualize

Oral Health   Quiet Alone

Today's Intention: Date:

What am I most proud of so far?

Celebrations/Concerns: Gratitude:

Opportunities:

"Good humor is the health of the soul, sadness is its poison."

- Philip Stanhope, 4th Earl of Chesterfield

My Mantra: Healing Habits:

Water   Movement
Meditation   Sleep
Clean Eating   Visualize
Oral Health   Quiet Alone

Date: _____

Where do I feel vulnerable? How is that give me positive motivation?

Gratitude:

Celebrations/Concerns:

Opportunities:

"Sponges grow in the ocean. That just kills me. I wonder how much deeper the ocean would be if that didn't happen."

　　　　　　　　　　　　　　- Steven Wright

Healing Habits:

Water   Movement
Meditation   Sleep
Clean Eating Visualize
Oral Health Quiet Alone

My Mantra:

Today's Intention: Date:

My best life in 5 years will feature . . . .

Celebrations/Concerns: Gratitude:

Opportunities:

Few of us ever live in the present. We are forever
anticipating what is to come or remembering what has
gone."

- Louis L Amour

My Mantra: Healing Habits:

    Water   Movement

    Meditation   Sleep

    Clean Eating   Visualize

    Oral Health   Quiet Alone

Date:

Define Hope.

Gratitude:

Celebrations/Concerns:

Opportunities:

"Without giving up hope-that there's somewhere better to be, that there's someone better to be-we will never relax with where we are or who we are."
- Pema Chödron When Things Fall Apart.

Healing Habits:

Water   Movement
Meditation   Sleep
Clean Eating   Visualize
Oral Health   Quiet Alone

My Mantra:

Today's Intention: Date:

What did I learn from a recent challenge?

Celebrations/Concerns: Gratitude:

Opportunities:

"Our present moment is a mystery that we are part
of. Here and now is where all the wonder of life lies
hidden. And make no mistake about it, to strive to live
completely in the present is to strive for what already
is the case."

- Wayne Dyer

My Mantra: Healing Habits:

Water   Movement
Meditation   Sleep
Clean Eating   Visualize
Oral Health   Quiet Alone

Date:

Today's Intention

What habit have you found to be most
effective with the least effort?

Gratitude:

Celebrations/Concerns:

Opportunities:

"True happiness, we are told, consists in getting out of
one's self, but the point is not only to get out - you
must stay out; and to stay out you must have some
absorbing errand."

- Henry James, Roderick Hudson

Healing Habits:

Water   Movement
Meditation   Sleep
Clean Eating   Visualize
Oral Health   Quiet Alone

My Mantra:

Today's Intention: Date:

Three things I look forward to daily are:

Celebrations/Concerns: Gratitude:

Opportunities:

"When you open your mind, you open new doors to new
possibilities for yourself and new opportunities to help
others."

- Roy T Bennett

My Mantra: Healing Habits:

Water   Movement
Meditation   Sleep
Clean Eating   Visualize
Oral Health   Quiet Alone

Date: _____

I am fully confident in my ability to . . . .

Gratitude:

Celebrations/Concerns:

Opportunities:

"Self-kindness. Being warm and understanding toward ourselves when we suffer, fail, or feel inadequate, rather than ignoring our pain or flagellating ourselves with self-criticism."

- Brene Brown

Healing Habits:

Water   Movement
Meditation   Sleep
Clean Eating   Visualize
Oral Health   Quiet Alone

My Mantra:

Today's Intention: Date:

I find delight in .

Celebrations/Concerns: Gratitude:

Opportunities:

"To be more childlike, you don't have to give up being an
adult. The fully integrated person is capable of being
both an adult and a child simultaneously. Recapture the
childlike feelings of wide-eyed excitement, spontaneous
appreciation, cutting loose, and being full of awe and
wonder at this magnificent universe."

- Wayne Dyer

My Mantra: Healing Habits:

Water   Movement
Meditation   Sleep
Clean Eating   Visualize
Oral Health   Quiet Alone

Date: _____

My top three priorities are:

Gratitude:

Celebrations/Concerns:

Opportunities:

"We may have fears about the future because we
don't know how it's going to turn out, and these worries
and anxieties keep us from enjoying being here now."
                                    - Thich Nhat Hanh

Healing Habits:

Water   Movement
Meditation   Sleep
Clean Eating   Visualize
Oral Health   Quiet Alone

My Mantra:

Today's Intention: Date:

An ideal day would look like:

Celebrations/Concerns: Gratitude:

Opportunities:

"You may say I'm a dreamer, but I'm not the only one. I
hope someday you'll join us. And the world will live as
one."

- John Lennon

My Mantra: Healing Habits:

Water   Movement
Meditation   Sleep
Clean Eating   Visualize
Oral Health   Quiet Alone

Date: Today's Intention

I experience self-compassion most often
when I . . . .

Gratitude: Celebrations/Concerns:

                                    Opportunities:

I think the foundation of everything in my life is wonder.
                                    - Alice Walker

Healing Habits: My Mantra:

   Water   Movement
   Meditation   Sleep
   Clean Eating   Visualize
   Oral Health   Quiet Alone

Today's Intention: Date:

One dream I've carried for a long time is

Celebrations/Concerns: Gratitude:

Opportunities:

"When we love, we always strive to become better than
we are. When we strive to become better than we
are, everything around us becomes better too."
                                                    - Paulo Coelho

My Mantra: Healing Habits:
                                                Water   Movement
                                                Meditation   Sleep
                                                Clean Eating   Visualize
                                                Oral Health   Quiet Alone

Date: _____

I admire . . . .

Gratitude:

Celebrations/Concerns:

Opportunities:

"It's really a wonder that I haven't dropped all my ideals, because they seem so absurd and impossible to carry out. Yet I keep them because in spite of everything, I still believe that people are really good at heart."
                    - Anne Frank, The Diary of a Young Girl

Healing Habits:

Water   Movement
Meditation   Sleep
Clean Eating   Visualize
Oral Health   Quiet Alone

My Mantra:

Today's Intention: Date:

I can do hard things. One challenge I recently
conquered is . . . .

Celebrations/Concerns: Gratitude:

Opportunities:

"You cannot swim for new horizons until you have
courage to lose sight of the shore."
                                        - William Faulkner

My Mantra: Healing Habits
                                           Water   Movement
                                           Meditation   Sleep
                                           Clean Eating   Visualize
                                           Oral Health   Quiet Alone

303

Date:

Consider a plan that didn't work out as you have first hoped, what gifts have you found that you had not considered?

Gratitude:

Celebrations/Concerns:

Opportunities:

"The meaning I picked, the one that changed my life:
Overcome fear, behold wonder."

~ Richard Bach

Healing Habits:

Water   Movement
Meditation   Sleep
Clean Eating   Visualize
Oral Health   Quiet Alone

My Mantra:

Today's Intention: Date:

My top 10 hopes for my best life are . . .

Celebrations/Concerns: Gratitude:

Opportunities:

"Life's under no obligation to give us what we expect."
- Margaret Mitchell

My Mantra: Healing Habits:
                                                    Water   Movement
                                                    Meditation   Sleep
                                                    Clean Eating   Visualize
                                                    Oral Health   Quiet Alone

Date: _____

Today i hope for . . . .

Gratitude:

Celebrations/Concerns:

Opportunities:

"Maybe everyone can live beyond what they're capable of."

- Markus Zusak

Healing Habits:

Water   Movement
Meditation   Sleep
Clean Eating   Visualize
Oral Health   Quiet Alone

My Mantra:

306

Today's Intention: Date:

Music is a powerful attitude adjustment tool, what
music feels right today?

Celebrations/Concerns: Gratitude:

Opportunities:

"Throw your dreams into space like a kite, and you do
not know what it will bring back, a new life, a new
friend, a new love, a new country."

- Anais Nin

My Mantra: Healing Habits:
                                                    Water   Movement
                                                    Meditation   Sleep
                                                    Clean Eating   Visualize
                                                    Oral Health   Quiet Alone

Date:

I choose love, today that means . . .

Gratitude: Celebrations/Concerns:

                                         Opportunities:

"You can cut all the flowers but you cannot keep
Spring from coming."
                              - Pablo Neruda

Healing Habits: My Mantra:

   Water   Movement
   Meditation   Sleep
   Clean Eating   Visualize
   Oral Health   Quiet Alone

End of Month Check In

1. How do you feel physically? What needs attention? What has improved?

2. What is your level of self-compassion? What can you do to support deeper self-compassion? What is working right now? What needs focus?

3. What is your level of connection to yourself and others? Can you be of service to others in a positive manner? What is working? What needs focus?

Changing Habits

Old Habit

New Habit

New Action

Affirmation

The Gift of Non-Attachment

ISSUE

LEVEL OF IMPORTANCE

_____

_____

DATE

PERSONAL / PROFESSIONAL

_____

_____

I WONDER

This exercise can transform your anxiety levels about outcome, from fear to peace, to recognize that you cannot control the outcome of the situation. You can manage your reaction to it and make choices that will influence the impact on your life. Notice the difference in your _feelings_ with each as you list your concerns.

I'm afraid that . .

_____

_____

_____

_____

_____

_____

_____

_____

_____

I wonder if . . .

_____

_____

_____

_____

_____

_____

_____

_____

Connection

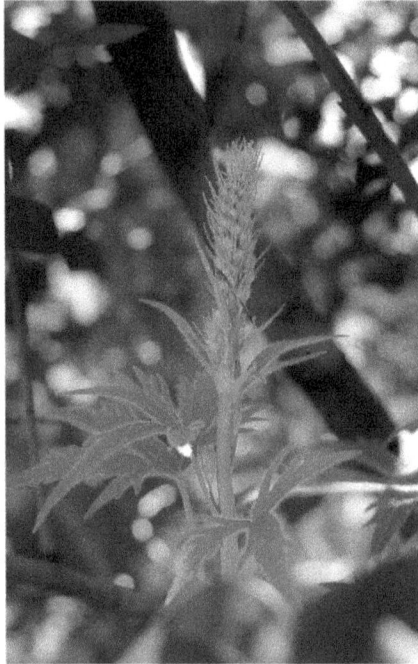

"When you love someone, you do not love
them all the time, in exactly the same
way, from moment to moment."
                    ~ Anne Morrow Lindbergh

Book: *Judgement Detox: Release the Beliefs That Hold You Back From Living A Better Life* by Gabrielle Bernstein

"In 2007, the "one that got away" sent me an email."

What does it mean to hold space for another person? It means that we are willing to walk alongside another person in whatever journey they're on without judging them, making them feel inadequate, trying to fix them, or trying to impact the outcome. When we hold space for another person, we open our hearts, offer unconditional support, and let go of judgment and control. ~ Heather Plett

In 2007, the "one that got away" sent me an email. After 22 years, Tom's marriage had ended, and he wondered if I would be interested in reconnecting. I had been in love with Tom since I was 18 years old. I introduced my children to the music he and I had listened to together during our last summer in college. We had both endured heartbreaks in the 30 years since we'd been in love, and we were cautious. I asked him to read seminal books on the topic. I had been single for nearly 20 years, so I knew what I was looking for and was done playing emotional mind games with less-than-worthy suitors. I was ready for a mutually respectful relationship, maintaining my independence while honoring his, sharing intimacy and joy as we share our lives together. Today, we incorporate balance, awareness, and acceptance within our relationship, offering one another support as needed.

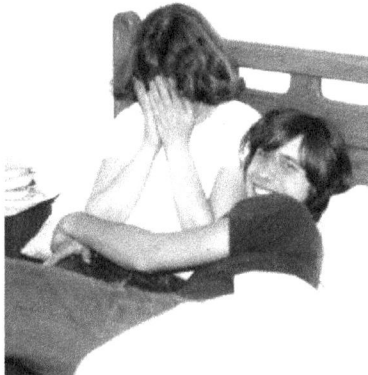

Other strong friendships that last through time have also been a huge part of my healing journey. I have had amazing support over the last 3 years from life-long friends and some that I met while recovering from my many health challenges in the last six years.

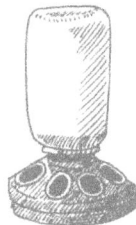

Connection and positive support have played as big a role in my transformation as healing interventions have. I have an incredible team now that I trust explicitly. The team I have been with for the last three years has become a part of my tribe.

Trustworthy personal support and medical teams are increasingly essential as we age. As our bodies mature, it becomes more and more important to build mutually respectful relationships with friends and medical professionals that understand our health priorities and the type of care we are most comfortable with. Have you got close friends and medical professionals that you can trust? I would like to urge you to garner meaningful support as you transform your life.

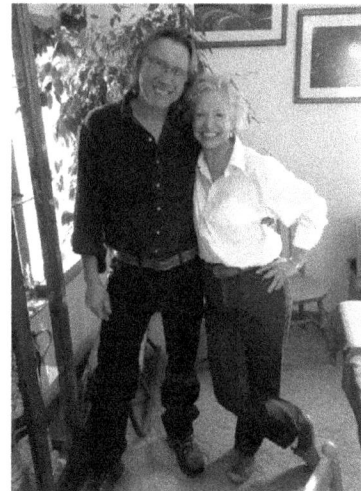

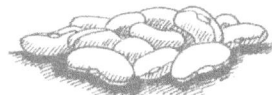

"Anything or anyone that asks you to be other than yourself is not holy, but it trying only to fill it's own need."

- Mark Nepo

Date:

Who am I through the eyes of compassion?

Gratitude:

Celebrations/Concerns:

Opportunities:

"Love does not consist in gazing at each other but in looking outward together in the same direction."
- Antoine de Saint-Exupery

Healing Habits:

Water   Movement
Meditation   Sleep
Clean Eating   Visualize
Oral Health   Quiet Alone

My Mantra:

Today's Intention: Date:

What do I want with connections to others?

Celebrations/Concerns: Gratitude:

Opportunities:

"I basically started performing for my mother, going,
'Love me!' What drives you to perform is the need for
that primal connection. When I was little, my mother
was funny with me, and I started to be charming and
funny for her, and I learned that by being entertaining
you make a connection with another person."
                                            - Robin Williams

My Mantra: Healing Habits:
                                                    Water   Movement
                                                    Meditation   Sleep
                                                    Clean Eating   Visualize
                                                    Oral Health   Quiet Alone

315

Date:

How can i be of service to others?

Gratitude:

Celebrations/Concerns:

Opportunities:

"When you love someone, you do not love them all the time, in exactly the same way, from moment to moment. "

- Anne Morrow Lindbergh

Healing Habits:

Water   Movement
Meditation   Sleep
Clean Eating   Visualize
Oral Health   Quiet Alone

My Mantra:

Today's Intention: Date:

What is my most cherished relationship today?

Celebrations/Concerns: Gratitude:

Opportunities:

"If you truly love someone, your love sees past their
humanness"

- Michael A. Singer

My Mantra: Healing Habits:

Water   Movement
Meditation   Sleep
Clean Eating   Visualize
Oral Health   Quiet Alone

Date: _____

Who supports my transformation efforts
most positively?

Gratitude:

Celebrations/Concerns:

Opportunities:

"Surround yourself with only people who are going to
lift you higher."
- Oprah Winfrey

Healing Habits:

Water   Movement
Meditation   Sleep
Clean Eating   Visualize
Oral Health   Quiet Alone

My Mantra:

Today's Intention: Date:

I know that a friendship is good when I can

Celebrations/Concerns: Gratitude:

Opportunities:

"In my own life I know that my state of cheerfulness
is a reliable gauge of my level of spiritual enlightenment
at that moment. The more cheerful, happy, contented,
and satisfied I am feeling, the more aware I am of my
deep connection to Spirit."

                                                    - Wayne Dyer

My Mantra: Healing Habits:

                                    Water   Movement
                                    Meditation   Sleep
                                    Clean Eating   Visualize
                                    Oral Health   Quiet Alone

My ideal romantic relationship looks like . . .

Gratitude:

Celebrations/Concerns:

Opportunities:

"The practice of forgiveness is our most important contribution to the healing of the world"
- Marianne Williamson

Healing Habits:

Water   Movement
Meditation   Sleep
Clean Eating   Visualize
Oral Health   Quiet Alone

My Mantra:

Today's Intention: Date:

My ideal friendship looks like .

Celebrations/Concerns: Gratitude:

Opportunities:

"The second agreement Don't take anything personally.
When you are immune to the opinions and actions of
others, you won't be the victim of needless suffering"
                                    - Don Miguel Ruiz

My Mantra: Healing Habits:
                                        Water   Movement
                                        Meditation   Sleep
                                        Clean Eating   Visualize
                                        Oral Health   Quiet Alone

Date:

Today's Intention:

My best quality as a friend is . . . .

Gratitude:

Celebrations/Concerns:

Opportunities:

"Sometimes the rewards of risk don't leave us wrecked. Sometimes we find our passion, our purpose, courage, connection, and comfort. Every good thing in our lives is a direct result of risk."

‐ Glennon Doyle

Healing Habits:

Water   Movement
Meditation   Sleep
Clean Eating   Visualize
Oral Health   Quiet Alone

My Mantra:

Today's Intention: Date:

I treat myself with the same gentle kindness I would
treat my child

Celebrations/Concerns: Gratitude:

Opportunities:

"A power struggle collapses when you withdraw your
energy from it. It cannot continue without your
intention to manipulate and control. When your intention
is to observe your inner process, everything else
changes. Power struggles become uninteresting to you
when you change your intention from winning to
learning about yourself."

- Gary Zukav and Linda Francis

My Mantra: Healing Habits:

                                                        Water   Movement
                                                        Meditation   Sleep
                                                        Clean Eating   Visualize
                                                        Oral Health   Quiet Alone

Date: _____

Today I will share gratitude

Gratitude:

Celebrations/Concerns:

Opportunities:

"Until we have seen someone's darkness, we don't really
know who they are. Until we have forgiven someone's
darkness, we don't really know what love is."
- Marianne Williamson

Healing Habits:

Water   Movement
Meditation   Sleep
Clean Eating   Visualize
Oral Health   Quiet Alone

My Mantra:

Today's Intention: Date:

i am a good friend and it shows when

Celebrations/Concerns: Gratitude:

Opportunities:

"The third agreement. Don't make assumptions. Find the
courage to ask questions and to express what you
really want. Communicate with others as clearly as you
can to avoid misunderstandings, sadness and drama."
                                          - Don Miquel Ruiz

My Mantra: Healing Habits:
                                                  Water   Movement
                                                  Meditation   Sleep
                                                  Clean Eating   Visualize
                                                  Oral Health   Quiet Alone

I am grateful for the kindness of others.
Today I will make an effort to be kind to a
stranger.

Gratitude:

Celebrations/Concerns:

Opportunities:

"As connected as we are with technology, it's also
removed us from having to have human connection,
made it more convenient to not be intimate."
- Sandra Bullock

Healing Habits:

My Mantra:

Water   Movement
Meditation   Sleep
Clean Eating   Visualize
Oral Health   Quiet Alone

Today's Intention: Date:

The best decision I've made in life is . . . .

Celebrations/Concerns: Gratitude:

Opportunities:

"True friendship is like sound health, the value of it is seldom known until it is lost."

- Charles Caleb Colton

My Mantra: Healing Habits:

Water   Movement
Meditation   Sleep
Clean Eating   Visualize
Oral Health   Quiet Alone

I can create a tribe around me that
supports healing I will look for those who . . .

Gratitude:

Celebrations/Concerns:

Opportunities:

"The biggest disease today is not leprosy or
tuberculosis, but rather the feeling of being unwanted."
- Mother Teresa

Healing Habits:

Water   Movement
Meditation   Sleep
Clean Eating   Visualize
Oral Health   Quiet Alone

My Mantra:

Today's Intention: Date:

i take time alone to connect to my highest self.

Celebrations/Concerns: Gratitude:

Opportunities:

"Money doesn't mean anything to me. I've made a lot of
money, but i want to enjoy life and not stress myself
building my bank account. I give lots away and live
simply, mostly out of a suitcase in hotels. We all know
that good health is much more important."
                                                    - Keanu Reeves

My Mantra: Healing Habits:
                                       Water   Movement
                                       Meditation   Sleep
                                       Clean Eating   Visualize
                                       Oral Health   Quiet Alone

Date: _____

Today's Intention: _____

I can make intelligent decisions when I take time alone to consider all possibilities. Today I will consider . . .

Gratitude:

Celebrations/Concerns:

Opportunities:

"If you would live long, open your heart."
- Bulgarian Proverb

Healing Habits:

Water   Movement
Meditation   Sleep
Clean Eating   Visualize
Oral Health   Quiet Alone

My Mantra:

Today's Intention: Date:

I am a creative problem solver. I love exploring
various options/outcomes. One recent issue I
handled well is . . . .

Celebrations/Concerns: Gratitude:

Opportunities:

"Home is where love resides, memories are created,
friends always belong, and laughter never ends."
                                        - Unknown

My Mantra: Healing Habits:
                                            Water   Movement
                                            Meditation   Sleep
                                            Clean Eating   Visualize
                                            Oral Health   Quiet Alone

I can maintain my own identity and share time with others.

Gratitude:

Celebrations/Concerns:

Opportunities:

"In my deepest, darkest moments, what really got me through was a prayer. Sometimes my prayer was 'Help me.' Sometimes a prayer was 'Thank you.' What I've discovered is that intimate connection and communication with my creator will always get me through because I know my support, my help, is just a prayer away."

- Iyanla Vanzant

Healing Habits:

Water   Movement
Meditation   Sleep
Clean Eating   Visualize
Oral Health   Quiet Alone

My Mantra:

Today's Intention: Date:

My communication within relationships is

Celebrations/Concerns: Gratitude:

Opportunities:

"The magic thing about home is that it feels good to
leave, and it feels even better to come back."
                    - Wendy Wunder, The Probability of Miracles

My Mantra: Healing Habits:
                                              Water   Movement
                                              Meditation   Sleep
                                              Clean Eating   Visualize
                                              Oral Health   Quiet Alone

333

Date:

I connect with honesty and openness

Gratitude:

Celebrations/Concerns:

Opportunities:

"Success means we go to sleep at night knowing that our talents and abilities were used in a way that served others."

- Marianne Williamson

Healing Habits:

Water   Movement
Meditation   Sleep
Clean Eating   Visualize
Oral Health   Quiet Alone

My Mantra:

Today's Intention: Date:

My favorite person is . . .

Celebrations/Concerns: Gratitude:

Opportunities:

                                "Loneliness is proof that your innate search for
                                connection is intact".
                                                            - Martha Beck.

My Mantra: Healing Habits:
                                                    Water   Movement
                                                    Meditation   Sleep
                                                    Clean Eating   Visualize
                                                    Oral Health   Quiet Alone

335

I can grow when I am alone.

Gratitude:

Celebrations/Concerns:

Opportunities:

"When you understand that being connected to others
is one of life's greatest joys, you realize that life's best
comes when you initiate and invest in solid relationships."
— John C. Maxwell

.

Healing Habits:

Water   Movement
Meditation   Sleep
Clean Eating   Visualize
Oral Health   Quiet Alone

My Mantra:

Today's Intention: Date:

i value mutual respect in relationships. I feel most
respected when .

Celebrations/Concerns: Gratitude:

Opportunities:

"Let us be grateful to people who make us happy, they
are the charming gardeners who make our souls
blossom"

- Marcel Proust

My Mantra: Healing Habits:
                                                 Water   Movement
                                                 Meditation   Sleep
                                                 Clean Eating   Visualize
                                                 Oral Health   Quiet Alone

Date: _____

I choose to spend time with those who are positive. My most positive connection is . . .

Gratitude:

Celebrations/Concerns:

Opportunities:

"Stay away from people with tiny minds and tiny thoughts and start hanging out with people who see limitless possibility as the reality. Surround yourself with people who act on their big ideas, who take action on making positive change in the world and who see nothing as out of their reach"

- Jen Sincero

Healing Habits:

Water   Movement
Meditation   Sleep
Clean Eating   Visualize
Oral Health   Quiet Alone

My Mantra:

Today's Intention: Date:

With whom do I need to set boundaries? I can set
boundaries as I need to.

Celebrations/Concerns: Gratitude:

Opportunities:

"There's love for your parents, your family, your
spouse, your partner, your friends, but the nature of
the connection you have with your child, there's nothing
like it. It has its own character and it's so serious and
so powerful, and so it's a prism through which I see
everything."

- Annette Bening

My Mantra: Healing Habits:
                                                   Water   Movement
                                                   Meditation   Sleep
                                                   Clean Eating   Visualize
                                                   Oral Health   Quiet Alone

Date: _____

Today's Intention: _____

I value honesty in relationships, I can always count on . . . .

Gratitude:

Celebrations/Concerns:

Opportunities:

"Communication is merely an exchange of information, but connection is an exchange of our humanity."
- Sean Stephenson

Healing Habits:

Water   Movement
Meditation   Sleep
Clean Eating   Visualize
Oral Health   Quiet Alone

My Mantra:

Today's Intention: Date:

i don't take things personally. i know that others'
behavior is a reflection of their own understanding
and perception.

Celebrations/Concerns: Gratitude:

Opportunities:

"Good communication is as stimulating as black coffee
and just as hard to sleep after."
                    - Anne Morrow Lindbergh, Gift from the Sea

My Mantra: Healing Habits:
                                             Water   Movement
                                             Meditation   Sleep
                                             Clean Eating   Visualize
                                             Oral Health   Quiet Alone

I have a clear sense of what I need to maintain as private and what to share.

Gratitude:

Celebrations/Concerns:

Opportunities:

"I believe that we have a huge problem with the water in America. We don't want to make that connection that these chemicals, at varying levels, in our water supplies, over time, is, in fact, related to our disease process. And it concerns me greatly."

　　　　　　　　　　　　　　　　- Erin Brockovich

Healing Habits:

Water   Movement
Meditation   Sleep
Clean Eating Visualize
Oral Health Quiet Alone

My Mantra:

Today's Intention: Date

How do i show my personal value?

Celebrations/Concerns: Gratitude:

Opportunities:

"The person that we will become in five years is
defined by the people that we spend time with today
and the books we read today."

- Jay Shetty

My Mantra: Healing Habits:

Water   Movement
Meditation   Sleep
Clean Eating   Visualize
Oral Health   Quiet Alone

End of Month Check In

1. How do you feel physically? What needs attention? What has improved?

2. What is your level of self-compassion? What can you do to support deeper self-compassion? What is working right now? What needs focus?

3. What is your level of connection to yourself and others? Can you be of service to others in a positive manner? What is working? What needs focus?

Changing Habits

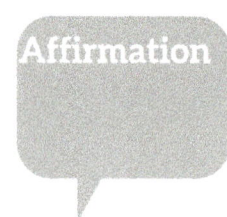

Old Habit

New Habit

New Action

Affirmation

Tame Emotional Responses

Negative Emotional Response

Situation?

Lightening or Thunder?

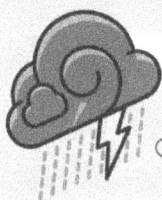

Common Negative Thoughts

- Do you see patterns or triggers that repeat themselves?
- Are there certain words, tones of voice, or sensory inputs that trigger an instant anger response?

Common Positive Thoughts

- Are you more tolerant in different settings, with different people, or at different times of day?
- If you have a difficult conversation, can you find a physically and emotionally safe time and place to do so?

Is the information I've received correct? Is is true? Can I trust the resources of information?

- How confident are you with the source of your information?
- Is there an agenda to the type of information that is being shared?
- Can you check with another source?

Positive Emotional Response

Situation?

Blue Skies and Sunny

Am I blaming, judging, or too invested in being *right*?
Have I considered other points of view?

Are you getting signals that tell you to **STOP AND PAY ATTENTION?**

- Anger, blame, righteous indignation and rage are often signs of fear or unresolved issues.
- Use them to remind you to look at the situation deeper or from a different angle.
- Can you approach the situation with curiosity, kindness or an open mind?
- Is there another way to see the issue?

What is the best possible outcome?

True Self

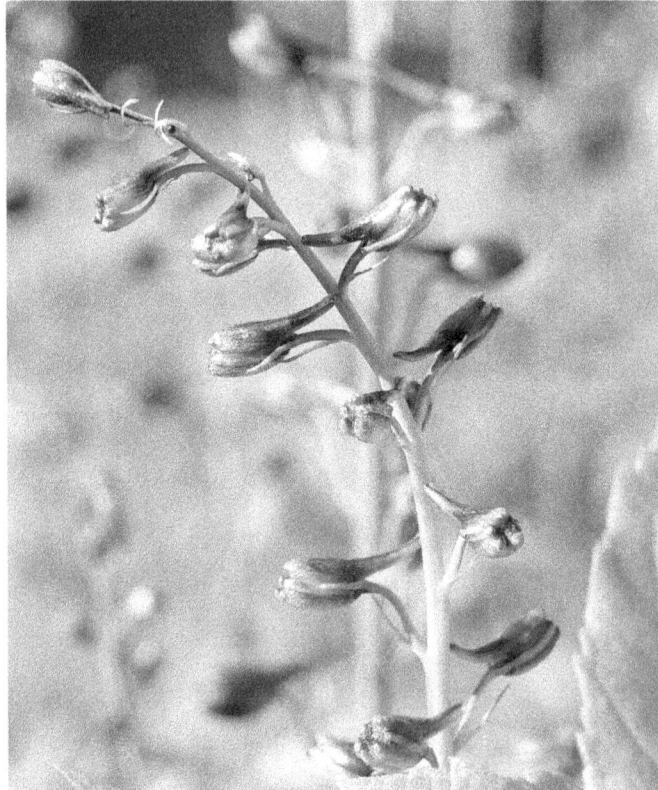

"Under all the thought and feelings lies the wisest, most complete version of yourself and it is your job to uncover it."

~ Jamie Bertini & John Kalinowski

Book: *The Untethered Soul* by Michael Singer

"My True Self is my own personal built-in barometer.."

An entire series of books could be written about one's True Self. Suffice it to say, I would like to be respectful of the magnitude of the topic yet succinct enough to reflect the core understanding of who we are essentially and how we connect to one another in meaningful ways. This self-understanding is synchronist with mindfulness in its most complete sense. It's a kind of "sixth sense," the knowing beyond knowing, a convicting source of inspiration and transformation. My work in developing my True Self provides autonomous direction but yields to the wisdom of others as well. I have learned to listen to that small voice within for my Truth, as evidenced by last year's misdiagnosed 9-month pregnancy!

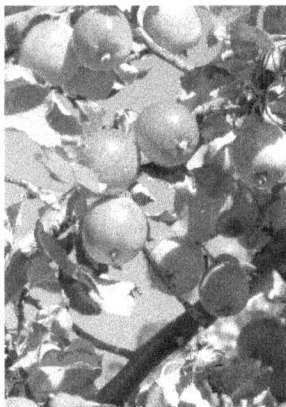

This exercise of arranging squiggles on paper has taught me an incalculable amount about myself, about my True Self. It has confirmed the validity of that voice within as the articulator of who I really am as a strong, capable, significant woman with life's experience as my ultimate teacher. This book is the product of reflecting upon my own True Self. I depend on It to reflect my values as a woman and my communion with humanity. Through meditative journaling, my True Self has gained a voice, and through the process of self-discovery, that small voice has gained strength.

My True Self is my own personal built-in barometer, my moral compass that guides me through life's travails. The internal and external direction, however, needs to be balanced and held in check. Too often in life, I have deferred to other people's best interests at the expense of my own. My True Self has a way of warning me against this, and it is up to me to pay attention to those warnings.

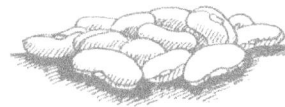

Don't believe everything you think. I never could figure out what that bumper sticker meant. Now I have fully embraced it. Is the thought a weed or a seed? Thoughts and emotions are like diaphanous clouds - morphing and changing constantly - observe them and let go of that which is not necessary.

In this process, I've discovered my "original blueprint," who I was meant to be. I've come to enjoy spending time every day with my True Self, which is the source of inner wisdom about my motives and desires as well as those of others. I find answers when I spend time with Her. She's always just a quiet nudge away, a constant companion, my Dearest Friend.

I would like to encourage you to get to know and spend time with your True Self, to garner wisdom about your inner workings and those of the world. That quiet voice within is always ready to speak when given a chance. It is best articulated when surrounded by silence. It will speak to you through meditation and journaling. I believe that as you write your journal you will find direction from your still, small voice that leads you deeper into your glorious Self.

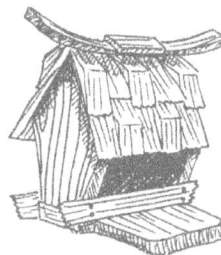

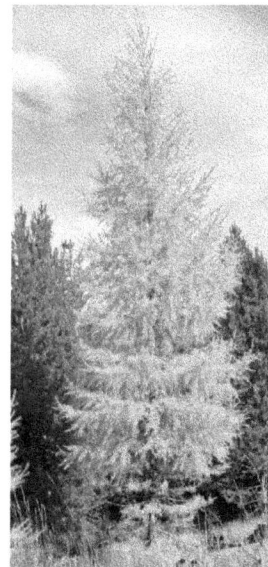

Date: _____

Who am I at my deepest core?

Gratitude:

Celebrations/Concerns:

Opportunities:

"Women need solitude in order to find again the true essence of themselves."
　　　- Anne Morrow Lindbergh, Gift from the Sea

Healing Habits:

Water　　　　　Movement
Meditation　　Sleep
Clean Eating　Visualize
Oral Health　　Quiet Alone

My Mantra:

348

Today's Intention: Date:

What do I want most?

Celebrations/Concerns: Gratitude:

Opportunities:

"What we do see depends mainly on what we look
for... In the same field the farmer will notice the
crop, the geologists the fossils, botanists the flowers,
artists the coloring, sportsmen the cover for the
game. Though we may all look at the same things, it
does not all follow that we should see them"

- John Lubbock

My Mantra   Healing Habits:

                                          Water   Movement
                                          Meditation   Sleep
                                          Clean Eating   Visualize
                                          Oral Health   Quiet Alone

Date:

How can I be of service to myself and others?

Gratitude:

Celebrations/Concerns:

Opportunities:

"To me, faith is not a public allegiance to a set of outer beliefs, but a private allegiance to the inner knowing. I stopped believing in the middlemen or hierarchy between me and God."

— Glennon Doyle

Healing Habits:

Water   Movement
Meditation   Sleep
Clean Eating   Visualize
Oral Health   Quiet Alone

My Mantra:

Today's Intention: Date:

What kind of life have I created?

Celebrations/Concerns: Gratitude:

Opportunities:

"The true voyage of self-discovery lies not in seeking
new landscapes but in having new eyes."

- Marcel Proust

My Mantra: Healing Habits:

Water   Movement
Meditation   Sleep
Clean Eating   Visualize
Oral Health   Quiet Alone

Date: _____

Do I feel comfortable seeing myself in a spiritual light?

Gratitude:

Celebrations/Concerns:

Opportunities:

"If we want to build the new, we must be willing to let the old burn. We must be committed to holding on to nothing but the truth. We must decide that if the truth inside us can burn a belief, a family structure, a religion, an industry - it should have become ashes yesterday."

- Glennon Doyle

Healing Habits:

Water   Movement
Meditation   Sleep
Clean Eating   Visualize
Oral Health   Quiet Alone

My Mantra:

352

Today's Intention: Date:

What does higher power mean to me?

Celebrations/Concerns: Gratitude:

Opportunities:

"God gave us memories so that we might have roses in
December"

- James M. Barrie

My Mantra   Healing Habits:

Water   Movement
Meditation   Sleep
Clean Eating   Visualize
Oral Health   Quiet Alone

What does my best self look like?

Gratitude:

Celebrations/Concerns:

Opportunities:

"Patience, patience, patience, is what the sea teaches. Patience and faith. One should lie empty, open, choice-less as a beach, waiting for a gift from the sea."

- Anne Morrow Lindbergh, Gift from the Sea

Healing Habits:

Water   Movement
Meditation   Sleep
Clean Eating   Visualize
Oral Health   Quiet Alone

My Mantra:

Today's Intention: Date:

How does my best self act on a daily basis?

Celebrations/Concerns: Gratitude:

Opportunities:

"The first agreement Be impeccable with your word.
Speak with integrity and say only what you mean.
Through the world you express your creative power.
Regardless of what language you speak, your intent
manifests throughout the world"

                                          - Don Miguel Ruiz

My Mantra: Healing Habits:

                    Water   Movement
                    Meditation   Sleep
                    Clean Eating   Visualize
                    Oral Health   Quiet Alone

Date: Today's Intention

What goals do I have as my best self?

Gratitude: Celebrations/Concerns:

                                         Opportunities:

"There is a huge amount of freedom that comes to
you when you take nothing personally."
                              - Don Miguel Ruiz

Healing Habits: My Mantra:

    Water   Movement
    Meditation   Sleep
    Clean Eating   Visualize
    Oral Health   Quiet Alone

Today's Intention: Date:

How do I see myself as the hero in my own story?

Celebrations/Concerns: Gratitude:

Opportunities:

"And I will ask the Father, and he will give you another
advocate to help you and be with you forever- the
Spirit of Truth. The world cannot accept him because
it neither sees him nor knows him"

- John 14 16 - 17 (NIV)

My Mantra: Healing Habits:
                                                      Water   Movement
                                                      Meditation   Sleep
                                                      Clean Eating   Visualize
                                                      Oral Health   Quiet Alone

Date:

What story have I told myself about my
health? Is there another lens from which to
view it?

Gratitude:

Celebrations/Concerns:

Opportunities:

"Spirituality is not about being perfect but about
aspiring to a life of heart-filled integrity. It is a
journey and not a destination. When we are spiritually
fit and balanced we are a powerfully exquisite blend
of human fallibility and divine perfection. It is this
dynamic tension that gives us our uniqueness, our
power to create and our compassion"
                                    - Caroline Reynolds

Healing Habits:

Water   Movement
Meditation   Sleep
Clean Eating   Visualize
Oral Health   Quiet Alone

My Mantra:

Today's Intention: Date:

What do I do on a daily basis that illuminates my best
self?

Celebrations/Concerns: Gratitude:

Opportunities:

"In the midst of winter, I finally learned that there was
within me, an invincible summer"

                                                    - Albert Camus

My Mantra: Healing Habits:
                                       Water   Movement
                                       Meditation   Sleep
                                       Clean Eating   Visualize
                                       Oral Health   Quiet Alone

Date:

Do i have a daily practice that i am not proud of?

Gratitude:

Celebrations/Concerns:

Opportunities:

"If someone does not want me it is not the end of the world. But if I do not want me, the world is nothing but endings."

- Nayyirah Waheed

Healing Habits:

Water   Movement
Meditation   Sleep
Clean Eating   Visualize
Oral Health   Quiet Alone

My Mantra:

Today's Intention: Date:

Within my most intimate relationship, I feel:

Celebrations/Concerns: Gratitude:

Opportunities:

"To accept the responsibility of being a child of God is
to accept the best that life has to offer"
                                        - Stella Terrill Mann

My Mantra: Healing Habits:

                                        Water   Movement
                                        Meditation   Sleep
                                        Clean Eating   Visualize
                                        Oral Health   Quiet Alone

Date: _____

Do I treat others as I want to be treated?

Gratitude: Celebrations/Concerns:

                                  Opportunities:

"Trust in yourself. Your perceptions are often far
more accurate than you are willing to believe."
                                  - Claudia Black

Healing Habits: My Mantra:

    Water   Movement
    Meditation   Sleep
    Clean Eating   Visualize
    Oral Health   Quiet Alone

Today's Intention: Date:

Today I will share a smile

Celebrations/Concerns: Gratitude:

Opportunities:

"Every form of art is another way of seeing the
world. Another perspective, another window. And
science -that's the most spectacular window of all.
You can see the entire universe from there."
                                          - Claudia Gray

My Mantra: Healing Habits

                                  Water   Movement
                                  Meditation   Sleep
                                  Clean Eating   Visualize
                                  Oral Health   Quiet Alone

Date: _____

Today's Intention: _____

My most important strength is . . . .

Gratitude:

Celebrations/Concerns:

Opportunities:

"Solitude matters, and for some people, it's the air they breathe."

— Susan Cain

Healing Habits:

Water
Meditation
Clean Eating
Oral Health

Movement
Sleep
Visualize
Quiet Alone

My Mantra:

Today's Intention: Date:

What is my favorite thing about myself?

Celebrations/Concerns: Gratitude:

Opportunities:

"Our culture made a virtue of living only as extroverts.
We discouraged the inner journey, the quest for a
center. So we lost our center and have to find it
again."

                                                    - Anais Nin

My Mantra: Healing Habits:
                                        Water   Movement
                                        Meditation   Sleep
                                        Clean Eating   Visualize
                                        Oral Health   Quiet Alone

What is one thing that I could improve that would take me closer to being my best self?

Gratitude:

Celebrations/Concerns:

Opportunities:

"Don't think of introversion as something that needs to be cured... spend your free time the way you like, not the way you think you're supposed to."
— Susan Cain

Healing Habits:

Water   Movement
Meditation   Sleep
Clean Eating Visualize
Oral Health Quiet Alone

My Mantra:

Today's Intention: Date:

What do I believe?

Celebrations/Concerns: Gratitude:

Opportunities:

"If we are always arriving and departing, it is also true
that we are eternally anchored. One's destination is
never a place but rather a new way of looking at
things."

- Henry Miller

My Mantra: Healing Habits:

                                                  Water   Movement
                                                  Meditation   Sleep
                                                  Clean Eating   Visualize
                                                  Oral Health   Quiet Alone

Is money an issue in my state of mind?

Gratitude:

Celebrations/Concerns:

Opportunities:

"..I want first of all - in fact, as an end to these
other desires - to be at peace with myself."
- Anne Morrow Lindbergh

Healing Habits:

Water   Movement
Meditation   Sleep
Clean Eating   Visualize
Oral Health   Quiet Alone

My Mantra:

Today's Intention: Date:

What are my values around time?

Celebrations/Concerns: Gratitude:

Opportunities:

"I'm an introvert... I love being by myself, love being
outdoors, love taking a long walk with my dogs and
looking at the trees, flowers, the sky"
                                            - Audrey Hepburn

My Mantra: Healing Habits:
                                              Water   Movement
                                              Meditation   Sleep
                                              Clean Eating   Visualize
                                              Oral Health   Quiet Alone

Date:

What are my values around food?

Gratitude:

Celebrations/Concerns:

Opportunities:

"The distance between insanity and genius is measured only by success"

- Ian Fleming

Healing Habits:

Water   Movement
Meditation   Sleep
Clean Eating Visualize
Oral Health Quiet Alone

My Mantra:

Today's Intention: Date:

What are my values about people different from
me?

Celebrations/Concerns: Gratitude:

Opportunities:

"Silence is only frightening to people who are
compulsively verbalizing."
                                    - William S. Boroughs

My Mantra: Healing Habits

                                        Water   Movement
                                        Meditation   Sleep
                                        Clean Eating   Visualize
                                        Oral Health   Quiet Alone

When was the last time you felt JOY in your body?

Gratitude:

Celebrations/Concerns:

Opportunities:

"In order to be open to creativity, one must have the capacity for constructive use of solitude. One must overcome the fear of being alone."

– Rollo May

Healing Habits:

Water   Movement
Meditation   Sleep
Clean Eating   Visualize
Oral Health   Quiet Alone

My Mantra:

Today's Intention: Date:

What is a quiet activity that brings you joy?

Celebrations/Concerns: Gratitude:

Opportunities:

"A happy life must be to a great extent a quiet life,
for it is only in an atmosphere of quiet that true joy
dares live."

- Bertrand Russell

My Mantra: Healing Habits:

Water   Movement
Meditation   Sleep
Clean Eating   Visualize
Oral Health   Quiet Alone

Date: _____

Today's Intention: _____

What form of movement brings you the most joy?

Gratitude:

Celebrations/Concerns:

Opportunities:

"Loving people live in a loving world. Hostile people live in a hostile world. Same world."

- Wayne W. Dyer

Healing Habits:

Water   Movement
Meditation   Sleep
Clean Eating   Visualize
Oral Health   Quiet Alone

My Mantra:

Today's Intention: Date:

What is your greatest strength?

Celebrations/Concerns: Gratitude:

Opportunities:

"Something amazing happens when we surrender and
just love. We melt into another world, a realm of
power already within us. The world changes when we
change. The world softens when we soften. The world
loves us when we choose to love the world."

- Marianne Williamson

My Mantra: Healing Habits:

Water   Movement
Meditation   Sleep
Clean Eating   Visualize
Oral Health   Quiet Alone

375

What is a weakness you could address that
would improve the quality of your life?

Gratitude:

Celebrations/Concerns:

Opportunities:

"The highest form of love is to be the protector of
another person's solitude."

- Rainer Maria Rilke

Healing Habits:

Water   Movement
Meditation   Sleep
Clean Eating   Visualize
Oral Health   Quiet Alone

My Mantra:

Today's Intention: Date:

What would you like more people to know about
you?

Celebrations/Concerns: Gratitude:

Opportunities:

"If the stars should appear but one night every
thousand years how man would marvel and adore"
                                    - Ralph Waldo Emerson

My Mantra   Healing Habits:
                                                       Water   Movement
                                                       Meditation   Sleep
                                                       Clean Eating   Visualize
                                                       Oral Health   Quiet Alone

Date: _____

I feel most myself when I . . .

Gratitude:

Celebrations/Concerns:

Opportunities:

"Without leaps of imagination or dreaming, we lose the excitement of the possibilities. Dreaming, after all, is a form of planning."

    - Gloria Steinem

Healing Habits:

Water   Movement
Meditation   Sleep
Clean Eating   Visualize
Oral Health   Quiet Alone

My Mantra:

End of Month Check In

1. How do you feel physically? What needs attention? What has improved?

2. What is your level of self-compassion? What can you do to support deeper self-compassion? What is working right now? What needs focus?

3. What is your level of connection to yourself and others? Can you be of service to others in a positive manner? What is working? What needs focus?

Changing Habits

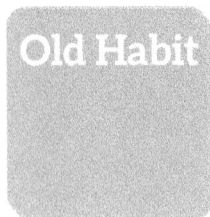

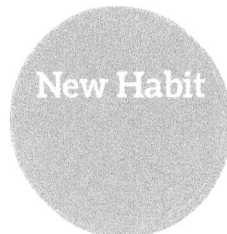

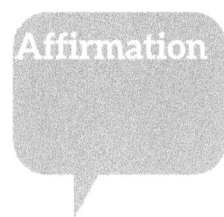

Old Habit

New Habit

New Action

Affirmation

PROBLEM SOLVING

Concern: Level Of Importance:

Date: Personal / professional

Central Issue:

Who is involved?

Does this affect my sense of safety?

- Have I experienced this before?
- IF a friend was in this situation how would I advise them?
- Is there a different way to look at this?
- Can I *listen* to the other person's point of view?
- Do I need some time to process this before I confront another?

- Does this affect my income?
- Does this affect my primary relationships?
- Does this affect my Health?
- Does This affect my sense of Self?

Possiblities   **Decision / Outcome**

Purpose

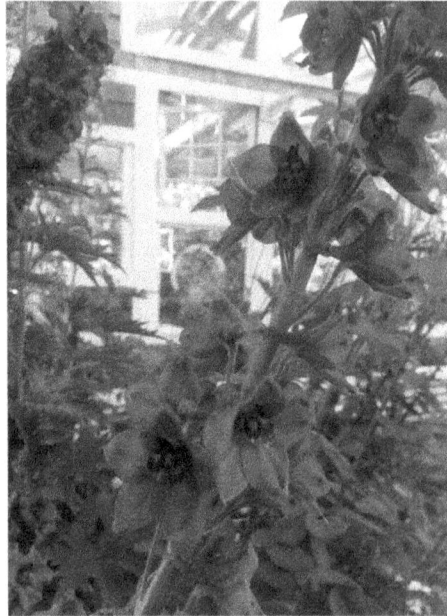

"To attain true inner freedom, you must be able to objectively watch your problems instead of being lost in them... Once you've made the commitment to free yourself of the scared person inside, you will notice that there is a clear decision point at which your growth takes place."

~ Michael A. Singer

Book: *The Art of Being: 101 Ways to Practice Purpose in Your Life*
by Dennis Merritt Jones, D.D.

"I was raised in a highly regimented environment."

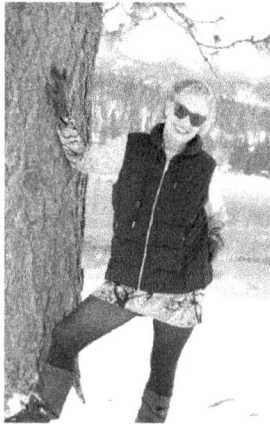

I was raised in a highly regimented environment. It's how my brain works best, so, in finding balance in my life, I have found a tool to use: structure. When I have a big project, I create a purpose statement to provide a structure for the project. I do this to keep me on track, to remind me of what I have set out to accomplish and why. It is a reminder, a path towards making my dream a reality. It's in black and white for me to check back when I'm not sure which step to take next.

Since my stroke, my brain behaves erratically, and, at times, it's scary. I use a purpose statement as a tool, a map to guide me along the way. A purpose statement lays out the path with a definite goal. It guides me on the step-by-step process of creating or becoming something better by living my best life. If I see later down the road that the original plan is not panning out the way I had envisioned, I have choices. I can allow for flow or flexibility, I can shift the format of the project, or decide to let it go and create a new purpose statement altogether. For others, having a much freer approach to things works. The important thing is to find what works best for you. Not getting attached to the outcome but staying open to seeing the path forward is essential.

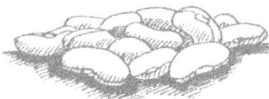

This journey through the FearLess journal has been yours and yours alone. My hope is that it has clarified your vision for your life and allowed you to put in place ways around life's challenges, interruptions, and the little messes that can accumulate along the way. Your purpose statement is equally yours and yours alone as well. YOU are the author of your life and the one to choose your own dreams. I encourage you to make your life exactly what you want it to be, to celebrate your True Self, and keep finding ways to make your best life a reality.

Wallowa County Finishing Salt

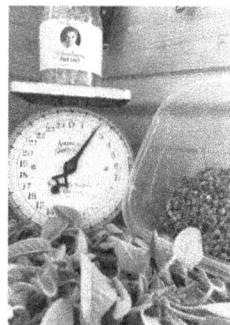

20 Juniper Berries

½ Cup Tightly Packed Fresh Sage Leaves

1 ½ cups coarse natural mineral or sea salt

4 garlic cloves finely minced

1 teaspoon freshly ground pepper

Mash the juniper berries with mortar and pestle - strip leaves from sage and rosemary and chop finely. Mince garlic and chop coarsely. Blend all ingredients and spread out of a cookie sheet and set out in a dry cool area for 3 or 4 days to dry out - you can cover it with a paper towel but it needs to breathe and dry out.

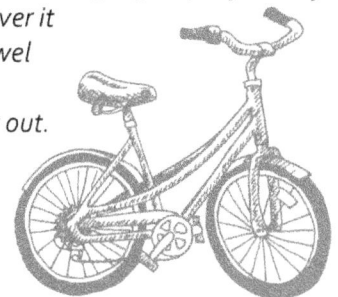

If you are one of the millions using Vitamin D supplements, and are also allergic or sensitive to WOOL, try vegan Vitamin D, most supplements are made with lanolin, a wool product.

Date: _____

Who am I in regards to style and substance?

Gratitude:

Celebrations/Concerns:

Opportunities:

"Our life is shaped by our mind; we become what we think. Suffering follows an evil thought as the wheels of a carts follow the oxen that draw it . . . joy follows a pure thought like a shadow that never leaves."

       - The Dhammadada

Healing Habits:

  Water   Movement
  Meditation   Sleep
  Clean Eating Visualize
  Oral Health   Quiet Alone

My Mantra:

Today's Intention: Date:

What do I want to accomplish today?

Celebrations/Concerns: Gratitude:

Opportunities:

"As we lose ourselves in the service of others we
discover our own lives and our own happiness."
                                        - Dieter F. Uchtdorf

My Mantra: Healing Habits:

Water   Movement
Meditation   Sleep
Clean Eating   Visualize
Oral Health   Quiet Alone

How can I be of service on a regular basis?

Gratitude:

Celebrations/Concerns:

Opportunities:

"...I want first of all - in fact, as an end to these
other desires - to be at peace with myself."
- Anne Morrow Lindbergh

Healing Habits:

Water   Movement
Meditation   Sleep
Clean Eating Visualize
Oral Health Quiet Alone

My Mantra:

Today's Intention: Date:

What do I love about my life?

Celebrations/Concerns: Gratitude:

Opportunities:

"Just as your car runs more smoothly and requires
less energy to go faster and farther when the wheels
are in perfect alignment, you perform better when
your thoughts, feelings, emotions, goals, and values are
in balance."

                                                    - Brian Tracy

My Mantra: Healing Habits:
                                            Water   Movement
                                            Meditation   Sleep
                                            Clean Eating   Visualize
                                            Oral Health   Quiet Alone

Date: Today's Intention:

Three things that have changed for the better
this year are . . . .

Gratitude: Celebrations/Concerns:

                                         Opportunities:

"If your life includes things you profess to hate, yet
you continue to do them anyway, that, too, indicates
self-betrayal . . . you can't possibly be living in concert
with who you were originally designed to be."
                                         - Dr. Phil McGraw

Healing Habits: My Mantra:

   Water   Movement
   Meditation   Sleep
   Clean Eating   Visualize
   Oral Health   Quiet Alone

Today's Intention: Date:

What parts of my life are working today?

Celebrations/Concerns: Gratitude:

Opportunities: "The truth is that you are responsible for what you think, because it is only at this level that you can exercise choice. What you do, comes from what you think."
                                                ~ Marianne Williamson

My Mantra: Healing Habits:

                                    Water   Movement
                                    Meditation   Sleep
                                    Clean Eating   Visualize
                                    Oral Health   Quiet Alone

Date: _____

What parts of my life are NOT working today?

Gratitude:

Celebrations/Concerns:

Opportunities:

"The truth is that you are responsible for what you think, because it is only at this level that you can exercise choice. What you do comes from what you think."

– Marianne Williamson

Healing Habits:

Water   Movement
Meditation   Sleep
Clean Eating   Visualize
Oral Health   Quiet Alone

My Mantra:

390

Today's Intention: Date:

What changes have I seen in my body and physical
health this year?

Celebrations/Concerns: Gratitude:

Opportunities:

"Before enlightenment, chop wood and carry
water ... after enlightenment, chop wood and carry
fire."

Ancient Buddist Wisdom

My Mantra: Healing Habits:

Water   Movement
Meditation   Sleep
Clean Eating   Visualize
Oral Health   Quiet Alone

I am learning to stay calm and accept
challenges as they appear.

Gratitude:

Celebrations/Concerns:

Opportunities:

"The best way to find yourself is to lose yourself in
the service of others."
- Mahatma Gandhi

Healing Habits:

My Mantra:

Water   Movement
Meditation   Sleep
Clean Eating   Visualize
Oral Health   Quiet Alone

Today's Intention: Date:

What changes have I witnessed in my relationships
this year?

Celebrations/Concerns: Gratitude:

Opportunities:

"The fourth agreement: Always do your best. Your
best is going to change from moment to moment.
Under any circumstance, always do your best, and you
will avoid self-judgement, self-abuse and regret."
                                        - Don Miguel Ruiz

My Mantra: Healing Habits:
                                            Water   Movement
                                            Meditation   Sleep
                                            Clean Eating   Visualize
                                            Oral Health   Quiet Alone

Date:

Today's Intention:

I can think clearly and process issues in a timely manner.

Gratitude:

Celebrations/Concerns:

"Learn to say no to demands, requests, invitations, and activities that leave you with no time for yourself. Until I learned to say no, and mean it, I was always overloaded by stress. You may feel guilty and selfish at first for guarding your down- time, but you'll soon find that you are a much nicer, more present, more productive person in each instance you do choose to say yes."

- Holly Mosier

Opportunities:

Healing Habits:

Water   Movement
Meditation   Sleep
Clean Eating   Visualize
Oral Health   Quiet Alone

My Mantra:

Today's Intention: Date:

When I focus on the positive . . .

Celebrations/Concerns: Gratitude:

Opportunities:

                                          "Mindfulness meditation doesn't change life. Life
                                          remains as fragile and unpredictable as ever.
                                          Meditation changes the heart's capacity to accept life
                                          as it is. It teaches the heart to be more
                                          accommodating not by beating it into submission, but
                                          by making it clear that accommodation is a gratifying
                                          choice."

                                                              - Sylvia Boorstein

My Mantra: Healing Habits:
                                             Water   Movement
                                             Meditation   Sleep
                                             Clean Eating   Visualize
                                             Oral Health   Quiet Alone

395

Date: _____

In what ways do I incorporate love into my life on a daily basis?

Gratitude:

Celebrations/Concerns:

Opportunities:

"Don't feel bad if people remember you only when they need you. Feel privileged that you are like a candle that comes to their mind when there is darkness."

- Bryce Adams

Healing Habits:

Water   Movement
Meditation   Sleep
Clean Eating   Visualize
Oral Health   Quiet Alone

My Mantra:

Today's Intention: Date:

What do I do daily to make sure I am focusing on the positive?

Celebrations/Concerns: Gratitude:

Opportunities:

"This is what one thirsts for, I realize, after the
smallness of the day, of work, of details, of intimacy -
even of communication, one thirsts for the magnitude
and universality of a night full of stars, pouring into
one like a fresh tide."
                    - Anne Morrow Lindbergh, Gift from the Sea

My Mantra: Healing Habits:
                              Water   Movement
                              Meditation   Sleep
                              Clean Eating   Visualize
                              Oral Health   Quiet Alone

Date:

Transformation brings change, I am
comfortable with change.

Gratitude:

Celebrations/Concerns:

Opportunities:

"We get upset at other people because they don't
meet our ideals of how they should act. Instead, try
accepting them for who they are, and recognizing
that, like you, they're imperfect and seeking
happiness and struggling with finding happiness.
They're doing their best. Accept them, smile, and enjoy
your time with this person."

- Leo Babauta

Healing Habits:

Water   Movement
Meditation   Sleep
Clean Eating   Visualize
Oral Health   Quiet Alone

My Mantra:

Today's Intention: Date:

What is my story?

Celebrations/Concerns: Gratitude:

Opportunities:

"Life's most persistent and urgent question is: What
are you doing for others?"

- Martin Luther King

My Mantra: Healing Habits:
                                                   Water   Movement
                                                   Meditation   Sleep
                                                   Clean Eating   Visualize
                                                   Oral Health   Quiet Alone

Date: _____

Today's Intention: _____

How has my story changed over this last year?

Gratitude:

Celebrations/Concerns:

Opportunities:

"The best way to capture moments is to pay attention. This is how we cultivate mindfulness. Mindfulness means being awake. It means knowing what you are doing."

— Jon Kabat-Zinn

Healing Habits:

Water   Movement
Meditation   Sleep
Clean Eating   Visualize
Oral Health   Quiet Alone

My Mantra:

400

Today's Intention: Date:

I see the world from a broad perspective.

Celebrations/Concerns: Gratitude:

Opportunities:

"While you'll feel compelled to charge forward it's
often a gentle step back that will reveal to you where
you and what you truly seek."

- Rasheed Ogunlaru

My Mantra: Healing Habits:

Water   Movement
Meditation   Sleep
Clean Eating   Visualize
Oral Health   Quiet Alone

Date: Today's Intention:

i have a belief system that blends well with my
personal values.

Gratitude: Celebrations/Concerns:

                                         Opportunities:

"Always ask yourself: "What will happen if I say
nothing?"
                        - Kamand Kojouri

Healing Habits: My Mantra:

   Water   Movement
   Meditation   Sleep
   Clean Eating   Visualize
   Oral Health   Quiet Alone

Today's Intention: Date:

i am open to compassion

Celebrations/Concerns: Gratitude:

Opportunities:

Earn your success based on service to others, not at
the expense of others"
                                                        - H. Jackson Brown Jr

My Mantra: Healing Habits:
                                                    Water   Movement
                                                    Meditation   Sleep
                                                    Clean Eating   Visualize
                                                    Oral Health   Quiet Alone

403

Date:

I am happiest when . . . .

Gratitude:

Celebrations/Concerns:

Opportunities:

"Suffering usually relates to wanting things to be
different from the way they are."

- Allan Lokos

Healing Habits:

Water   Movement
Meditation   Sleep
Clean Eating   Visualize
Oral Health   Quiet Alone

My Mantra:

Today's Intention: Date:

The last time i felt "freedom of movement"
was

Celebrations/Concerns: Gratitude:

Opportunities:

"Don't let a day go by without asking who you are.
each time you let a new ingredient to enter your
awareness"

- Deepak Chopra

My Mantra: Healing Habits:
                                                   Water   Movement
                                                   Meditation   Sleep
                                                   Clean Eating   Visualize
                                                   Oral Health   Quiet Alone

Date:

My goal is living vibrantly, today I can . . .

Gratitude:

Celebrations/Concerns:

"

Opportunities:

You have two hands. One to help yourself, the second
to help others."

- Audrey Hepburn

Healing Habits:

Water   Movement
Meditation   Sleep
Clean Eating   Visualize
Oral Health   Quiet Alone

My Mantra:

Today's Intention: Date:

I make decisions based on love when I...

Celebrations/Concerns: Gratitude:

Opportunities:

"It stands to reason that anyone who learns to live well
will die well. The skills are the same: being present in
the moment, and humble, and brave, and keeping a
sense of humor."

- Victoria Moran

My Mantra: Healing Habits:
                                             Water   Movement
                                             Meditation   Sleep
                                             Clean Eating   Visualize
                                             Oral Health   Quiet Alone

Date:

Today's Intention:

Is it true?

Gratitude:

Celebrations/Concerns:

Opportunities:

"Diversity is an aspect of human existence that cannot be eradicated by terrorism or war or self-consuming hatred. It can only be conquered by recognizing and claiming the wealth of values it represents for all."

– Aberjhani

Healing Habits:

Water
Meditation
Clean Eating
Oral Health

Movement
Sleep
Visualize
Quiet Alone

My Mantra:

Today's Intention: Date:

If I could have one do-over . . . .

Celebrations/Concerns: Gratitude:

Opportunities:

"As we encounter new experiences with a mindful and
wise attention, we discover that one of three things
will happen to our new experience: it will go away, it
will stay the same, or it will get more intense.
whatever happens does not really matter"
                                        - Jack Kornfield

My Mantra: Healing Habits:
                                            Water   Movement
                                            Meditation   Sleep
                                            Clean Eating   Visualize
                                            Oral Health   Quiet Alone

Date: _____

Today's Intention: _____

What habit have I worked hard to develop this year?

Gratitude:

Celebrations/Concerns:

Opportunities:

"To give real service, you must add something which cannot be bought or measures with money."
- Douglas Adams

Healing Habits:

Water	Movement
Meditation	Sleep
Clean Eating	Visualize
Oral Health	Quiet Alone

My Mantra:

Today's Intention: Date:

What habit do I need to change to achieve excellent
health?

Celebrations/Concerns: Gratitude:

Opportunities:

"Treat everyone you meet as if they were you"
                                              - Doug Dillon

My Mantra: Healing Habits:
                                              Water   Movement
                                              Meditation   Sleep
                                              Clean Eating   Visualize
                                              Oral Health   Quiet Alone

Date: Today's Intention:

What is one thing that throws me out of
balance?

Gratitude: Celebrations/Concerns:

                                         Opportunities:

"We too should make ourselves empty, that the great
soul of the universe may fill us with its breath."
                              - Lawrence Binyon

Healing Habits: My Mantra:

    Water   Movement
    Meditation   Sleep
    Clean Eating Visualize
    Oral Health Quiet Alone

Today's Intention: Date:

If I had more time I would . . . .

Celebrations/Concerns: Gratitude:

Opportunities:

"Love in action is service to the world"
                                    - Lynne Namka

My Mantra: Healing Habits:

                                        Water   Movement
                                        Meditation   Sleep
                                        Clean Eating   Visualize
                                        Oral Health   Quiet Alone

1. How do you feel physically? What needs attention? What has improved?

2. What is your level of self-compassion? What can you do to support deeper self-compassion? What is working right now? What needs focus?

3. What is your level of connection to yourself and others? Can you be of service to others in a positive manner? What is working? What needs focus?

Changing Habits

Old Habit

New Habit

New Action

Affirmation

Personal Purpose Statement:

A Guide to Living Your Best Life

Who Are YOU? Physically Emotionally Socially
Intellectually Spiritually Professionally?

What past successes have improved the quality of my life?
What are my strengths and weaknesses? What challenges do I have that
affect my opportunities?

What are my core values and how do they affect my life on a daily basis?
What are my current goals for all areas of health?
What is my hope for my future best life?

What are some practical considerations to be addressed as I transition to my
best life? How do my intentions affect the lives of those in my life?

What shape do I wan the rest of my life to take? Describe my ideal life?
What steps do I need to take with your body, mind and soul to achieve that
life?

Take as much time as you need this month to contemplate these questions.
Then, write them out clearly to use as a guide. Get creative and make it
beautiful so you can display it somewhere you will see it daily.

Transformation

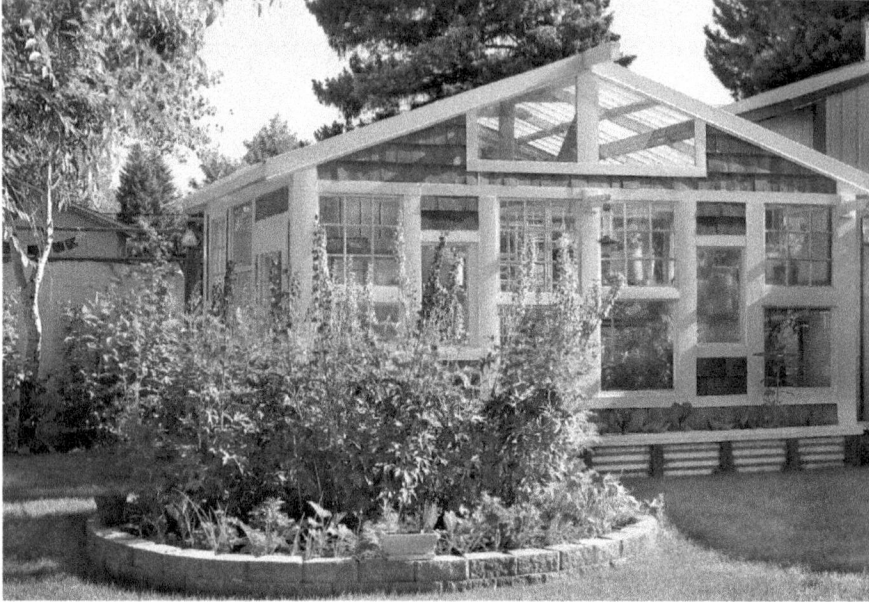

"There is a reason the sky gets dark at night. We were not meant to see everything all the time. We were meant to rest and trust, even in the darkness."

~Morgan Harper Nichols

Habit :
Awareness

Challenges in Western Medicine - Shifting the Healthcare
Paradigm: | Dr. Mimi Guarneri | TEDxAmericasFinestCity
Book: *Rituals for Transformation* by Briana Borten
and Dr. Peter Borten

"Transformation reminds me of a winter night's dream about planning my summer garden."

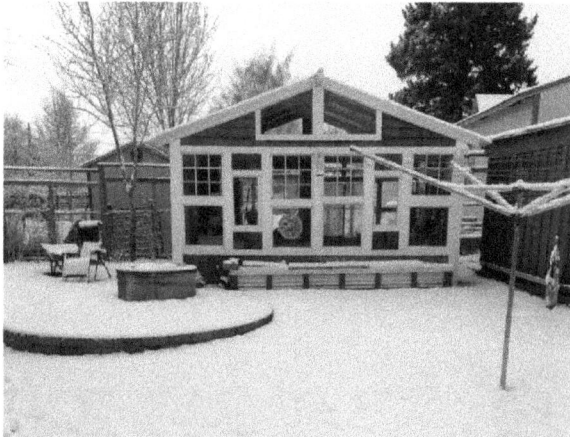

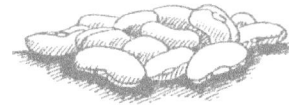

One of the most important tips I give clients: Check all pharmaceuticals and supplements for reactivity and side effects. Talk to your doctor about your current regime and reduce as much as possible.

Transformation reminds me of a winter night's dream about planning my summer garden. Paging through the seed catalogs and picking out next year's candidates and refusing the rejects is a lot like my transformation process. Yes, transformation is a lot like choosing the best seeds for our inner garden and rejecting the ones that just don't cut the mustard. In exploring the depths of my interior architecture, I've come to realize the need to declutter the unnecessary and repopulate with the necessary. For example, I've expanded my knowledge base by going back to school and becoming an integrative health coach. As I worked on getting myself healthy again, on a very deep level, I knew that my thought and belief systems were no longer helping me reach my full potential. I needed more. The primary purpose of hiring a health coach was to give me the opportunity to bring in some personalized fresh thinking. I knew that I'd taken myself as far as I could and I needed some outside thinking to support a new way of seeing life.

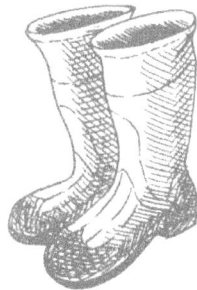

In many ways, transformation is a process of interior evolution, one shaped by all sorts of experiences and education.

Some of these have served me well, and some of the others have harmed me. Using meditation, self-exploration, journaling, and working closely with my coach have all been quite helpful. "Can I find inner peace and live my life fully and exactly how I want to?" The answer is YES. And yes, I can find inner peace if I am willing to undergo the process of editing the junk from my life. Ultimately, my forgiveness has liberated me from the prison of self-doubt and self-recrimination. It was the cornerstone of the blossoming that my coach led me to. What a relief!

You may have found some of the answers to your questions in this journal or in some of the books you've read. Only you can earn transformation, seeking the answers with passion will lead to your True Self! Take what works for you and keep it. If there is a belief system that does not work, change it. In truth, in the most ultimate sense of Eternal Truth, self-love, the kind that transforms us into the sacred creatures that we essentially are, is the only way to move forward toward health and overall well-being. So, here's the question: What do you need to discard so that you can transform into the You that you were intended to be?

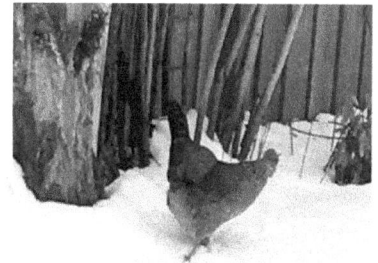

417

Date:

Who am I in my best life?

Gratitude:

Celebrations/Concerns:

The problem is not merely one of Woman and
Career, Woman and the Home, Woman, and
Independence. It is more basically: how to remain
whole in the midst of the distractions of life, how to
remain balanced, no matter what centrifugal forces
tend to pull one off center, how to remain strong,
no matter what shocks come in at the periphery and
tend to crack the hub of the wheel."
　　　Anne Morrow Lindbergh, Gift from the Sea

Opportunities:

Healing Habits:

Water   Movement
Meditation   Sleep
Clean Eating   Visualize
Oral Health   Quiet Alone

My Mantra:

Today's Intention: Date:

Who am I personally?

Celebrations/Concerns: Gratitude:

Opportunities:

"If you light a lamp for someone else it will also
brighten your path."

                                                    - Buddha

My Mantra: Healing Habits
                                              Water   Movement
                                              Meditation   Sleep
                                              Clean Eating   Visualize
                                              Oral Health   Quiet Alone

419

Date: _____

Today's Intention: _____

Who am I in my closest personal relationships?

Gratitude:

Celebrations/Concerns:

Opportunities:

"I do not think that I will ever reach a stage when I
say, "This is what I believe. Finished." What I believe is
alive and open to growth."

- Madeleine L'Engle

Healing Habits:

Water   Movement
Meditation   Sleep
Clean Eating   Visualize
Oral Health   Quiet Alone

My Mantra:

Today's Intention: Date:

Who am I professionally?

Celebrations/Concerns: Gratitude:

Opportunities:

"Let there be peace on earth, and let it begin with me."

- Romi M. Panlilio

My Mantra: Healing Habits:

Water   Movement
Meditation   Sleep
Clean Eating   Visualize
Oral Health   Quiet Alone

Date: Today's Intention:

What do I want?

Gratitude: Celebrations/Concerns:

                                         Opportunities:

"I don't think that anything happens by coincidence.
No one is here by accident. Everyone who crosses
our path has a message for us. Otherwise they
would have taken another path, or left earlier or
later. The fact that these people are here means
that they are here for some reason"..."
                              - James Redfield

Healing Habits: My Mantra:

    Water   Movement
    Meditation   Sleep
    Clean Eating   Visualize
    Oral Health   Quiet Alone

Today's Intention: Date:

What do I want for myself?

Celebrations/Concerns: Gratitude:

Opportunities:

"I slept and dreamt that life was joy. I awoke and saw
that life was service. I acted and behold, service was
joy."

- Rabindranath Tagore

My Mantra: Healing Habits:
                                                    Water   Movement
                                                    Meditation   Sleep
                                                    Clean Eating   Visualize
                                                    Oral Health   Quiet Alone

Date:

What do I want in my closest personal relationships?

Gratitude:

Celebrations/Concerns:

Opportunities:

"Each of us has a unique part to play in the healing of the world"

- Marianne Williamson, The Law of Divine Compensation: Mastering the Metaphysics of Abundance

Healing Habits:

Water   Movement
Meditation   Sleep
Clean Eating   Visualize
Oral Health   Quiet Alone

My Mantra:

Today's Intention: Date:

What do I want professionally?

Celebrations/Concerns: Gratitude:

Opportunities:

"Give a man health and a course to steer, and he'll
never stop to trouble about whether he's happy or
not."

- George Bernard Shaw

My Mantra: Healing Habits:

Water   Movement
Meditation   Sleep
Clean Eating   Visualize
Oral Health   Quiet Alone

Date: Today's Intention:

What do I need?

Gratitude: Celebrations/Concerns:

                                   Opportunities:

"If you really want to receive joy and happiness, then
serve others with all your heart. Lift their burden,
and your own burden will be lighter."
                        - Ezra Taft Benson

Healing Habits: My Mantra:

   Water   Movement
   Meditation   Sleep
   Clean Eating   Visualize
   Oral Health   Quiet Alone

Today's Intention: Date:

What do I need to feel happy?

Celebrations/Concerns: Gratitude:

Opportunities:

"Eat breakfast like a king, lunch like a prince, and
dinner like a pauper."

- Adelle Davis

My Mantra: Healing Habits
                                             Water   Movement
                                             Meditation   Sleep
                                             Clean Eating   Visualize
                                             Oral Health   Quiet Alone

Date:

Today's Intention:

What do I need to feel healthy?

Gratitude:

Celebrations/Concerns:

Opportunities:

"Happiness is the highest form of health."
- Dalai Lama

Healing Habits:

Water   Movement
Meditation   Sleep
Clean Eating   Visualize
Oral Health   Quiet Alone

My Mantra:

Today's Intention: Date:

What do i need to feel connected?

Celebrations/Concerns: Gratitude:

Opportunities:

"Eating healthy food fills your body with energy and
nutrients. Imagine your cells smiling back at you and
saying "Thank you!"."

- Karen Salmansohn

My Mantra: Healing Habits:

                                      Water   Movement
      Meditation   Sleep
      Clean Eating   Visualize
      Oral Health   Quiet Alone

Date:

What do I need to feel like I am making smart choices?

Gratitude:

Celebrations/Concerns:

Opportunities:

"Do your little bit of good where you are, its those little bits of good put together that overwhelm the world."

- Desmond Tutu

Healing Habits:

Water   Movement
Meditation   Sleep
Clean Eating   Visualize
Oral Health   Quiet Alone

My Mantra:

Today's Intention: Date:

What do i need to feel connected to my true self
or a higher power?

Celebrations/Concerns: Gratitude:

Opportunities:

"To be sensual, i think, is to respect and rejoice in the
force of life, of life itself, and to be present in all
that one does, from the effort of loving to the
breaking of bread."

                                                    - James Baldwin

My Mantra: Healing Habits:
                                            Water   Movement
                                            Meditation   Sleep
                                            Clean Eating   Visualize
                                            Oral Health   Quiet Alone

Date: _____

How can I be of service?

Gratitude:

Celebrations/Concerns:

Opportunities:

"The best way to find yourself is to lose yourself in the service of others."
- Mahatma Gandhi

Healing Habits:

Water   Movement
Meditation   Sleep
Clean Eating   Visualize
Oral Health   Quiet Alone

My Mantra:

Today's Intention: Date:

How can I practice better self-care?

Celebrations/Concerns: Gratitude:

Opportunities:

"Don't believe everything you think. Thoughts are just
that - thoughts"
    - Allan Lokos, Pocket Peace: Effective Practices
      for Enlightened Living

My Mantra: Healing Habits:
                                               Water   Movement
                                               Meditation   Sleep
                                               Clean Eating Visualize
                                               Oral Health Quiet Alone

Date: _____   Today's Intention: _____

What random act of kindness can I perform today?

Gratitude: Celebrations/Concerns:

                                    Opportunities:

"No man can be really free in bed with a woman who is not."

— Nancy Friday, My Secret Garden

Healing Habits: My Mantra:

Water   Movement
Meditation   Sleep
Clean Eating   Visualize
Oral Health   Quiet Alone

Today's Intention:

Date:

What is most important to me today?

Celebrations/Concerns:

Gratitude:

Opportunities:

"Respond, don't react.
Listen, don't talk.
Think, don't assume."
- Raji Lukkoor

My Mantra:

Healing Habits

Water   Movement
Meditation   Sleep
Clean Eating   Visualize
Oral Health   Quiet Alone

Date: _____

What do I need to feel safe?

Gratitude:

Celebrations/Concerns:

Opportunities:

"The best way to not feel hopeless is to get up and do something. Don't wait for good things to happen to you. If you go out and make some good things happen, you will fill the world with hope, you will fill yourself with hope."

— Barack Obama

Healing Habits:

Water   Movement
Meditation   Sleep
Clean Eating   Visualize
Oral Health   Quiet Alone

My Mantra:

Today's Intention: Date:

What do I need to feel loved?

Celebrations/Concerns: Gratitude:

Opportunities:

"Yoga practice can make us more and more sensitive
to subtler and subtler sensations in the body. Paying
attention to and staying with finer and finer
sensations within the body is one of the surest ways
to steady the wandering mind."

                                                    - Ravi Ravindra

My Mantra: Healing Habits:
                                                 Water   Movement
                                                 Meditation   Sleep
                                                 Clean Eating Visualize
                                                 Oral Health   Quiet Alone

What do I need to feel connected within my close relationships?

Gratitude:

Celebrations/Concerns:

Opportunities:

"It's good to have an end in mind but in the end what counts is how you travel."

- Orna Ross

Healing Habits:

Water
Meditation
Clean Eating
Oral Health

Movement
Sleep
Visualize
Quiet Alone

My Mantra:

Today's Intention: Date:

What do I need to feel connected in my community?

Celebrations/Concerns: Gratitude:

Opportunities:

"You are what you do, not what you say you'll do"
- Carl Gustav Jung

My Mantra: Healing Habits:
                                              Water   Movement
                                              Meditation   Sleep
                                              Clean Eating   Visualize
                                              Oral Health   Quiet Alone

Date: Today's Intention:

How can I incorporate moments of peace
and quiet into my day?

Gratitude:

Celebrations/Concerns:

Opportunities:

"Do the best you can until you know better. Then
when you know better, do better."
- Maya Angelou

Healing Habits:

Water   Movement
Meditation   Sleep
Clean Eating   Visualize
Oral Health   Quiet Alone

My Mantra:

Today's Intention: Date:

What can I do to incorporate a day of rest each
week?

Celebrations/Concerns: Gratitude:

Opportunities:

"There is a reason the sky gets dark at night. We
were not meant to see everything all the time. We
were meant to rest and trust, even in the darkness."
                              - Morgan Harper Nichols

My Mantra: Healing Habits:

                                        Water   Movement
                                        Meditation   Sleep
                                        Clean Eating   Visualize
                                        Oral Health   Quiet Alone

How can I incorporate service to others on a daily basis in my life?

Gratitude:

Celebrations/Concerns:

Opportunities:

"Breathe, Darling. This is just a chapter. It's not the whole story."

- S. C. Lourie

Healing Habits:

Water   Movement
Meditation   Sleep
Clean Eating   Visualize
Oral Health   Quiet Alone

My Mantra:

Today's Intention: Date:

Can I incorporate a day of service once a week
or month?

Celebrations/Concerns: Gratitude:

Opportunities:

"The best antidote I know for worry is work. The
best cure for weariness is the challenge of helping
someone who is even more tired. One of the great
ironies of life is this: He or she who serves almost
always benefits more than he or she who is served"
                                    - Gordon B. Hinckley

My Mantra: Healing Habits:
                                    Water   Movement
                                    Meditation   Sleep
                                    Clean Eating   Visualize
                                    Oral Health   Quiet Alone

Date:

Today's Intention:

What can I do on a daily basis to support acting from my highest self most of the time?

Gratitude:

Celebrations/Concerns:

Opportunities:

"Everything we do is infused with the energy with which we do it. If we're frantic, life will be frantic. If we're peaceful, life will be peaceful. And so our goal in any situation becomes inner peace."
- Marianne Williamson

Healing Habits:

Water   Movement
Meditation   Sleep
Clean Eating   Visualize
Oral Health   Quiet Alone

My Mantra:

Today's Intention: Date:

How can I forgive myself for moments when I act
without grace?

Celebrations/Concerns: Gratitude:

Opportunities:

When you reach a calm and quiet meditative state,
that is when you can hear the sound of silence'
                                              - Stephen Richards

My Mantra: Healing Habits:
                                                   Water   Movement
                                                   Meditation   Sleep
                                                   Clean Eating   Visualize
                                                   Oral Health   Quiet Alone

How can I best address fear and learn from it?

Gratitude:

Celebrations/Concerns:

Opportunities:

"Your own Self-Realization is the greatest service you can render the world."

- Ramana Maharshi

Healing Habits:

Water
Meditation
Clean Eating
Oral Health

Movement
Sleep
Visualize
Quiet Alone

My Mantra:

Today's Intention: Date:

What is the most important thing I can do to
improve my life?

Celebrations/Concerns: Gratitude:

Opportunities:

"You should never be afraid of revealing your true
colours. After all, what could be more beautiful than
who you really are. Sure, to some you may be a mess
of muddy dark browns or oil spill greens, but to
others, you'll sparkle blue like an ocean, you'll glitter
gold like a ring"

                                                    - Beau Taplin

My Mantra: Healing Habits:

         Water   Movement
         Meditation   Sleep
         Clean Eating   Visualize
         Oral Health   Quiet Alone

What is the most important thing I can do to improve the life of my significant personal relationships?

Gratitude:

Celebrations/Concerns:

Opportunities:

"The secret to finding the deeper level in the other is finding the deeper level in yourself, without finding it in yourself, you cannot see it in another".

- Eckhart Tolle

Healing Habits:

Water   Movement
Meditation   Sleep
Clean Eating   Visualize
Oral Health   Quiet Alone

My Mantra:

End of Month Check In

1. How do you feel physically? What needs attention? What has improved?

2. What is your level of self-compassion? What can you do to support deeper self-compassion? What is working right now? What needs focus?

3. What is your level of connection to yourself and others? Can you be of service to others in a positive manner? What is working? What needs focus?

Changing Habits

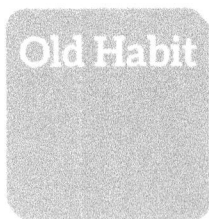

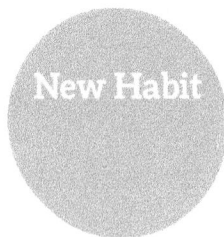

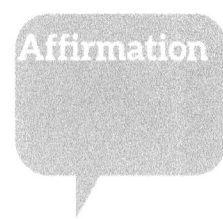

Old Habit

New Habit

New Action

Affirmation

Decision Making 101

Identify the Issue

Date

Give yourself time to
process.

Look at the issue from at
least 3 different angles.

Options

Positive / Negative
Outcomes

Ask Questions

Can this problem be re-framed?
        Best case scenario?
        Worst case scenario?
What would you decide if you
were already living your ideal
life?
If you knew you could not fail,
what would you decide?

Choose Among Your
Options

Take Action

Assess Outcome

◯ AMAZING

◯ GREAT

◯ GOOD

◯ OKAY

◯ BAD

Your Path Toward Courage

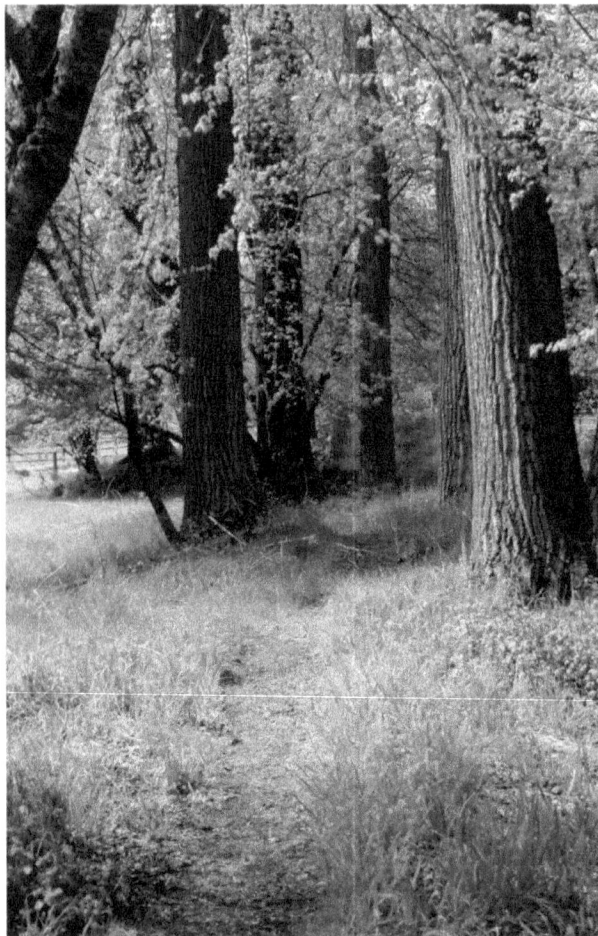

You have completed your journey towards courage in this *Blossom's FearLess* journal. You have done this on your own! You have done the hard work, you have dug deep, and have walked the path of compassion to your deepest Truest Self. I am so proud of you for taking the time and prioritizing yourself each day, starting your day off with your True Self, exploring, growing, learning, reframing old beliefs, and establishing firm healing habits that support your best health. It helps to have a daily ritual in which you spend quiet time alone, completely unplugged, and open to answers to your unspoken questions from your most essential core being. I am so proud of you for creating these anchor habits that refocus you daily on your life's purpose. You have created a pattern of commitment to your best Self.

A daily ritual of self-care, journaling, visualizing the day ahead, exploring words of wisdom, moving your body, checking in physically, and breathing new life into the new day all encourage you to blossom into the Self you were originally designed to be. Your life cannot be transformed with 3.5 minutes a day of rote journaling 5 items for which you are grateful. However, you can streamline your morning rituals by combining your healing habits into a schedule that works for you. You may divide these activities throughout your day. You can try audio recordings of your thoughts and things that you are grateful for, making note of the healing habits you have practiced. Moving your body in a daily yoga routine that incorporates checking in physically with deep breathing sets your objective for optimal health. The fact that you have carved out this much time this year for yourself is something to put into your celebration column. Taking the time to meditate and collect your thoughts, to set an intention for your day, to invite grace through gratitude, and to acknowledge your victories and concerns and the opportunities they may provide are all the best ways to begin the day. I hope you have blossomed through these practices.

Dedicating time for yourself each day is the one way to remain open to the answers you seek in your daily life. Consciously choosing love and releasing fear-based thoughts, messages, and situations on a daily basis are essential to a positive mindset. Maintaining a balance between your physical, emotional, social, intellectual, and spiritual health has become routine, and when you miss a day of movement, you recognize the beginning of clouded thinking. Using your healing habits tracker to monitor different health indicators is a useful tool to make sure you are well hydrated, have slept properly, and have maintained other self-care issues. Giving yourself the gift of time and space to take care of you before you are of service to others is the ultimate way to live your best life. Inviting grace by expressing gratitude completes the picture.

My wish for you is that you have found your purpose. My hope is that you can take the principals you have embraced on this journey and incorporate them into your days ahead to improve the quality of your day-to-day experience. I also hope that you have found in yourself a new best friend in your Self that always has the right answers. I hope that you have been able to embrace your bio-individuality and let go of trying to manage others' lives based on your own personal truth. I wonder what your future will look like as you live with positive intent and invite peace and quiet into your life.

This journal is just the start. I wish you peace and joy in every language.

Namaste -

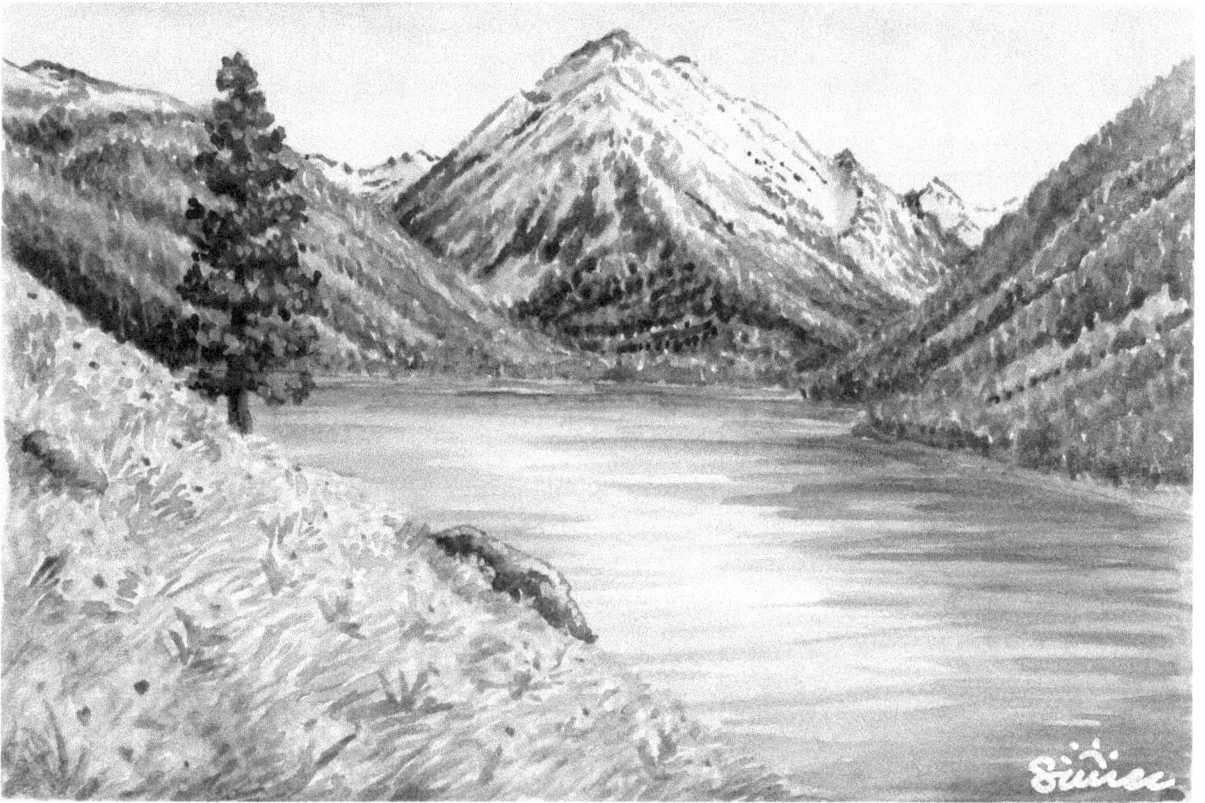

Acknowledgements

Writing a book has been a dream since I was very young. My stroke erased a lot of my cognitive and language abilities for a very long time. I didn't see how writing a book could even be possible, so I started this project knowing that there was much to learn. I have heaps of gratitude for my publishing team. We have worked well together to create a beautiful and therapeutic journal and transformation program. Our book is tough to fit into any one genre. It is first and foremost a program to help support balance and excellent health. It is, however, also a memoir of the last three years of my life, a self-help guide packed with resources to support living our best life. Finally, and perhaps most relevant, it is an artful book for you to write your story within. I have many to acknowledge in crafting this journal. I must first and foremost thank my husband, Tom, who has been so patient with stacks of books and papers everywhere for the last six months. Tom has given me the time and space to make a dream come true. I am truly lucky to have re-connected with him 12 years ago. He, too, is realizing his dream to be a graphic artist, and his photography and technical advice have been gentle and consistent throughout this project. My editor, George Boesger, has been amazingly generous with his time and brilliance. What a gift he has been throughout this process! I could not have done this without him. Any grammatic or style errors are all mine. Summer Derrickson has been the most amazing technical assistant. Consulting her watercolor art has been inspirational. Her enthusiasm and easy-going nature has been contagious and has made this collaboration one of the most rewarding professional experiences ever. I am also grateful to the Institute for Integrative Learning and the Launch Your Dream Book Class for offering this bonus class, enabling this dream to come to fruition. I've journaled since 5th grade, hoping to use these journals as research for a book. One gift of journaling has been the thought that my journey might someday help others, and with this book, I have had my dream become tangible. I set out to create a project of gratitude and service and have been able to accomplish both with this book. I hope that you find joy within.

Recommendations

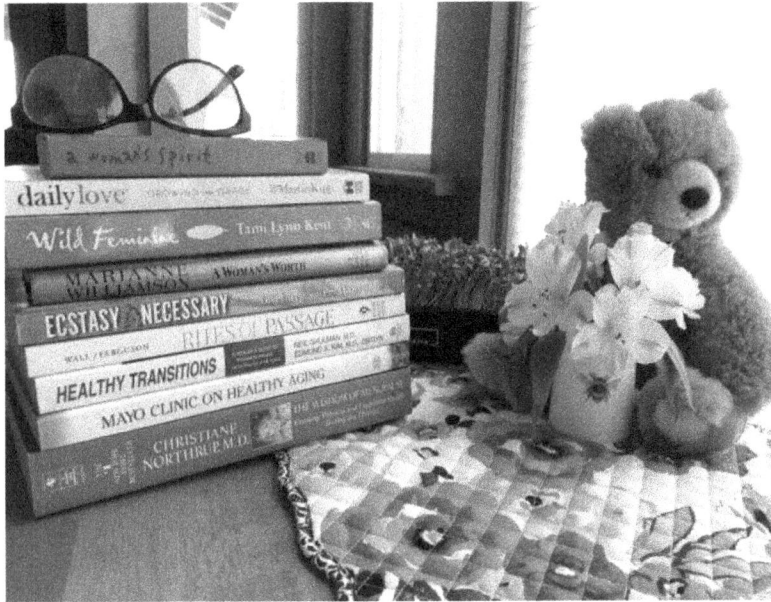

Choose Love

Let Go Of Fear

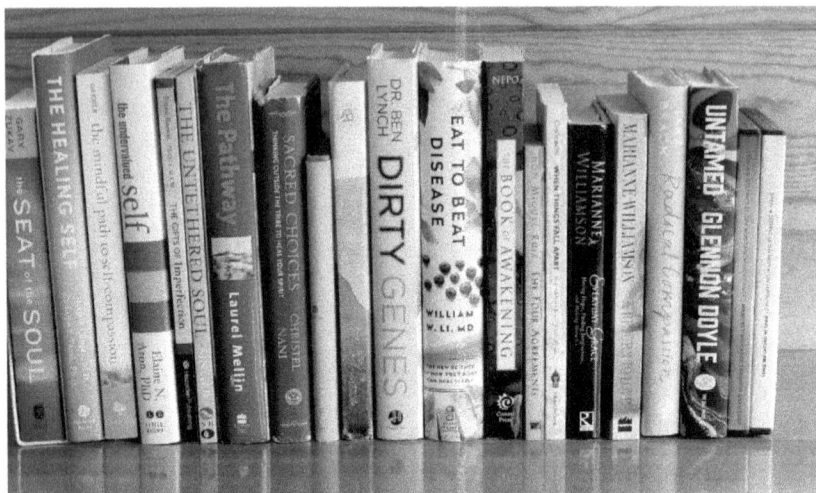

The Pathway Laurel Mellin
Alexander and Terrible, Horrible Very Bad, No Good, Day Judith Viorst
A Woman's Worth Marianne Williamson
Brave Enough Cheryl Strayed
A Course In Miracles: 365 Miracles Mind Media Press
The Secret Garden Frances Hodgson Burnett
Embracing Uncertainty Susan Jeffers, Ph,D,
The Four Agreements Don Miquel Ruiz
The Lanuage of Love Gary Smalley and John Trent

Love Your Body

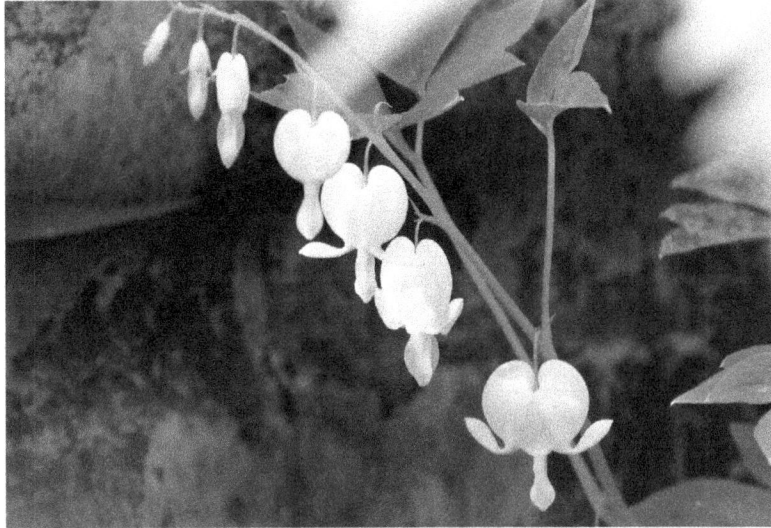

I Quit Sugar: Your Complete 8-Week Detox Program   Sarah Wilson
All Around the World Cookbook   Sheila Lukins
Eat to Beat Disease William W. Li M.D.
A Bad Case of Stripes   David Shannon
It Starts with Food   Melissa Hartwig, Dallas Hartwig
TedTalk: *"Can We Eat To Starve Cancer?"* William W. Li M.D.
Dirty Genes Ben Lynch M.D.
The Science of Natural Healing, Great Courses Mimi Guarneri M.D.
It Was Me All Along Andie Mitchell
"Yoga With Adriane" YouTube Adriane Mishler
Mapping Human History Steve Olson

Mindfulness

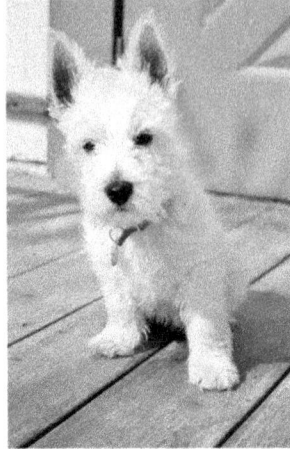

The Mindfulness Path to Self-Compassion   Christopher K. Germer Ph.D
TedX Nashville: *"Self-Transformation through Mindfulness"* Dr. David Vago
Wherever You Go, There You Are Jon Kabat-Zinn
The Three Questions   Jon J. Muth
Sacred Choices: Thinking Outside the Tribe Christel Nani
I am Peace: A Book of Mindfulness Susan Verde, Peter H. Reynolds
Rising Strong Brene' Brown
Music Album: *"Janis Ian: Between the Lines"* Janis Ian
Coach Yourself To Success   Talane Meidaner
Kneaded Touch Mark and Luemily Pugh
Mindfulness Magazine
Moonshine Glass Art (Meditation River Egg)

Compassion

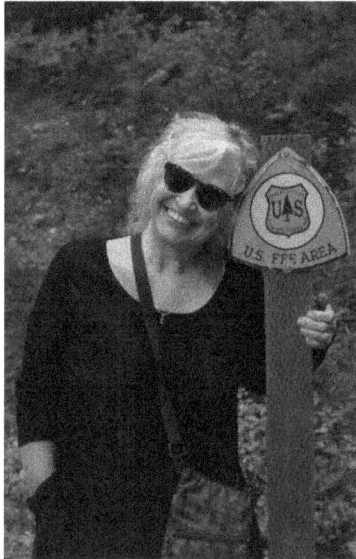

Radical Compassion Tara Brach
The Highly Sensitive Parent Elaine N. Aron, Ph.D.
Winter Garden Kristen Hannah
The Body Keeps Score Bessel van der Kolk, M.D.
The World According to Mr. Rogers Fred Rogers
Better than Before Gretchen Rubin
The Blue Day Book: A Lesson in Cheering Yourself Up Bradly Trevor Greive
Girl Wash Your Face Rachel Hollis
The Exquisite Risk Mark Nepo
Becoming Michelle Obama
The Indomitable Gertrude Green Max W. Hammonds

Gratitude Invites Grace

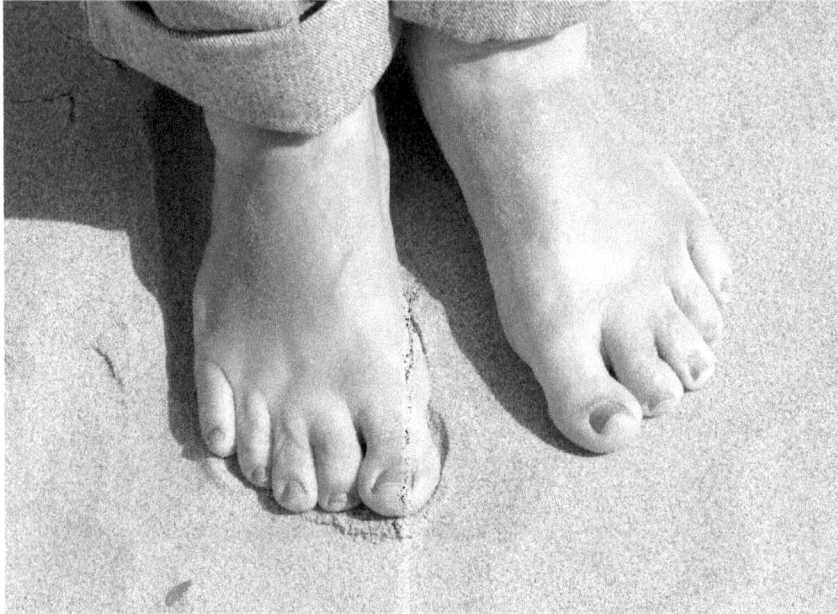

The Gifts of Imperfection Brene' Brown
Everyday Grace Marianne Willamson
Gratitude Manifests Grace," 21-day Meditation
Deepak Chopra, Oprah Winfrey
Gratitude   Louie Schwartzberg
The Book Of Joy   Dali Lama, Desmond Tutu
Grace Not Perfection Emily Lee
Discernment Beth Ann Estock
Finding Your Way Home: A Soul Survival Kit   Melody Beattie
Moonshine Glass Art Enterprise, Oregon

Courage, Curiosity, and Grit

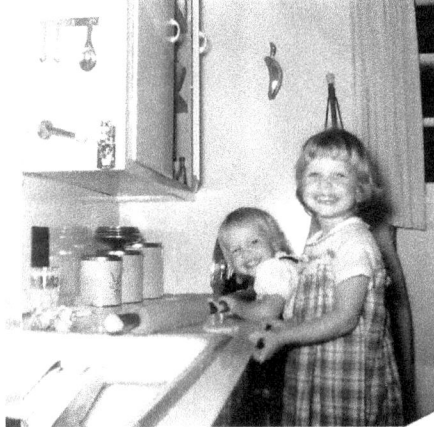

Untamed Glennon Doyal

Freedom Is An Inside Job Zainab Salbi

Fear: Essential Wisdom For Getting Through The Storm Thich Nhat Hanh

Feel The Fear and Do It Anyway Susan Jeffers Ph.D.

Daring Greatly Brene' Brown

Bridge to Terabithia Katherine Paterson, Donna Diamond

I Think I Am Louise L. Hay & Kristina Tracy

Grit: The Power of Passion and Perseverance Angela Duckworth

A Time To Forgive Darold Bigger

Heal Your Body

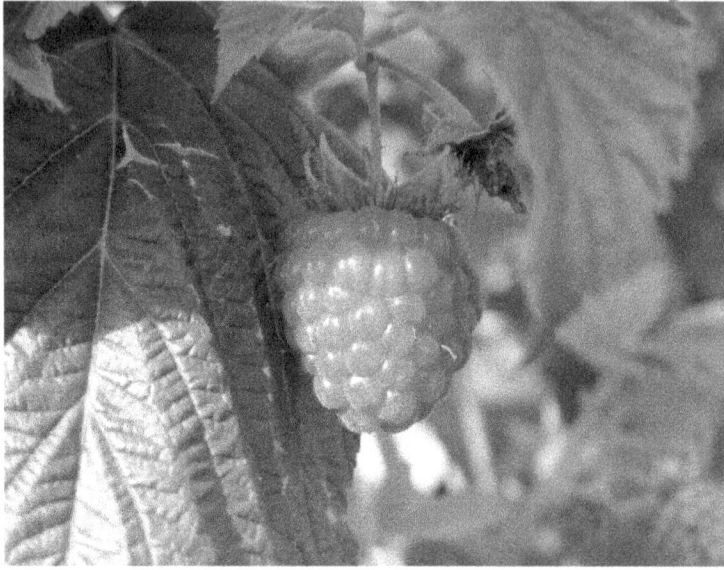

The Healing Self   Deepak Chopra, Rudolph E. Tanzi, Ph.D.
The Wahls Protocol Terry Wahls
TedX Iowa City: *Minding Your Mitochondria* Terry Wahls M.D.
Liver Rescue   Anthony Williams
108 Pearls to Awaken Healing Potential   Mimi Guarnei M.D.
Feeding You Lies   Vani Hari
The Immune System Recovery Plan   Susan Blum, M.D., Michele Bender Toxic: *Heal Your Body* Neil Nathan M.D.
The Complete Guide to Fasting   Jason Fung M.D., and Jimmy Moore
The Aging Brain Timothy R. Jennings M.D.
Institute of Integrative Nutrition

Wonder and Hope

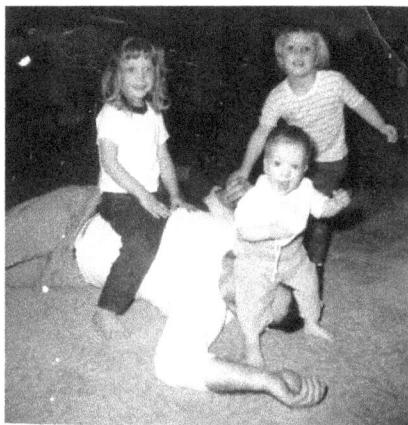

Wired for Healing: Remapping the Brain   Anne Hopper
Dynamic Neural Retraining,
RetrainingTheBrain.com   Anne Hopper
Wonder   R. J. Palacio
Ever Changing Perspective Gareth Michael
The Book of Awakening   Mark Nepo
"Hope in Uncertain Times," 21-day Meditation
Deepak Chopra, Oprah Winfrey
A Gradual Awakening Stephen Levine
The Power of NOW Echart Tolle
Belonging: Remembering Ourselves Home   Toko-pa Turner
You Can Heal Your Life   Louise L. Hay
YouTube: "Seeds, Weeds & Intention"   Russel Brand

Connection

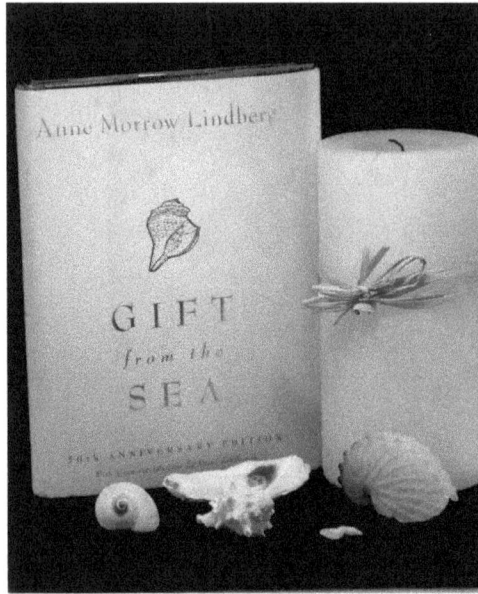

Think Like a Monk   Jay Shetty
"Creating Peace from the Inside Out"
21-day Meditation
Deepak Chopra, Oprah Winfrey
Growing Up Again   Jean Illsley Clarke, Connie Dawson
Gift from the Sea   Anne Morrow Lindbergh
The Dance of Connection Harriet Learner, Ph.D.
The Gift of Change Marianne Williamson
Wild Feminine   Tami Lynn Kent
The Velveteen Rabbit   Marjorie Williams
Personality Plus Florence Littauer
Irregular People Joyce Landorf
Outlander Series Diana Gabaldon

True Self

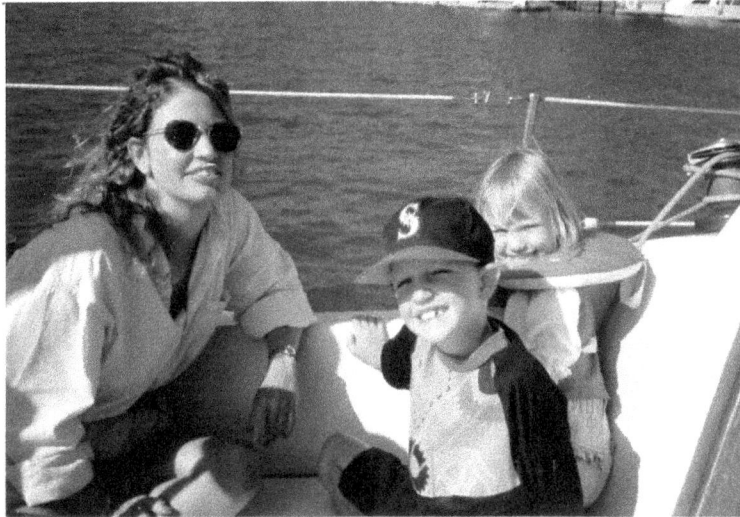

The Untethered Soul Michael A. Singer
The Mastery of Love   Don Miquel Ruiz
The Undervalued Self Elaine N. Aron, Ph.D.
The Art of Ritual Renee Beck, Sydney Barbara Metrick
The Neurobiology of We Danial J Siegel
The Seat of The Soul Gary Zukav
Judgment Detox   Gabrielle Bernstein
The Incident at Hawks Hill Allen W. Eckert
Finding Your Authentic Self Jennifer Ladouceur
Every Day Holy Melanie Shankle
Finding your own North Star Martha Beck

Purpose

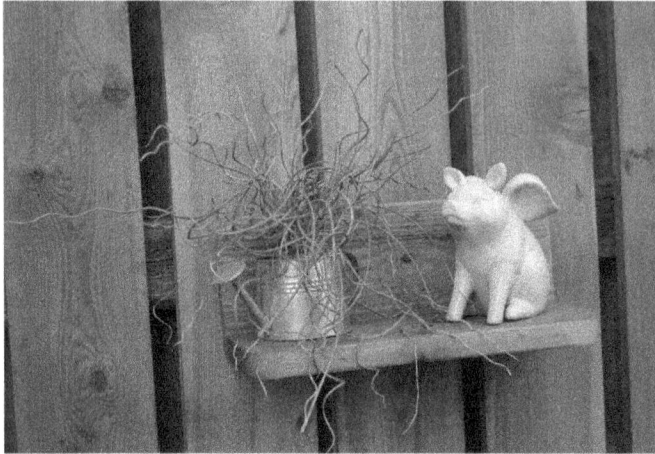

The Art of Being Dennis Merritt Jones, DD
The Last Lecture Randy Pausche and Jeffery Zaslow
All About Love Bell Hooks
Brain Wash: Detox Your Mind David & Austin Perlmutter, M.D.,
Kristin Loberg
Change Your Brain, Change Your Life Danial Amen M.D
Attached Amir Levine, M.D. and Rachel S.F. Heller, M.A.
Critical Conversations Kerry Patterson,
Joseph Grenny, Ron McMillan, Al SwizlerIt's
Within You Rabbi Aryeh Weinstein, Irene S. Cohen, Ph.D.
The Artist's Way Julia Cameron
Mountain Monarch Herbals @GoldenMonarchHerbals

Transformation

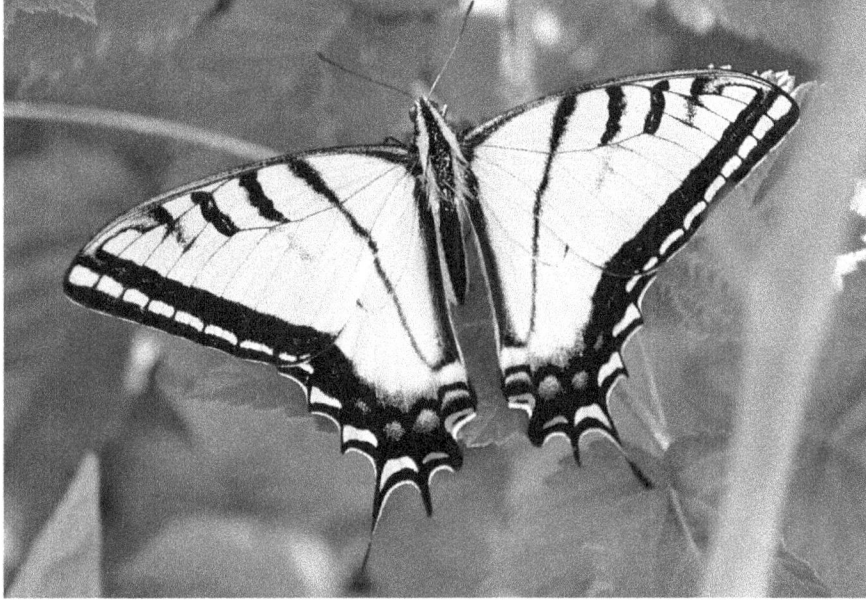

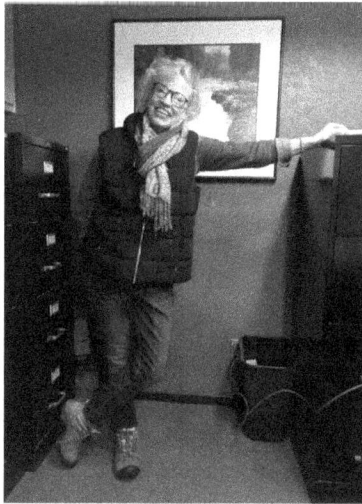

Graduation Day Institute of Integrative Nutrition

This book was inspired, in part, by my experience at the Institute for Integrative Nutrition(R) (IIN) where I receive my training in holistic wellness and health coaching. I initially went to educate myself on exactly how my body works in regards to food, healing, and integrated wellness and balance. I got that and so much more. IIN offers a truly comprehensive Health Coach Training Program that invites students to explore the things that are the most nourishing to them. From the physical aspects of nutrition and eating whole foods that work best for each individual, to the concept of Primary Food - the idea that everything in life, including our spirituality, career, relationships, and fitness contributes to our inner and outer health. IIN helped me reach optimal health and balance. This inner journey unleashed the passion that compels me to share what I have learned and inspire others. Beyond personal health, IIN offers training in health coaching as well as business and marketing. Students who choose to pursue the field professional complete the program equipped with the communication skills and branding knowledge they need to create a fulfilling career encouraging and supporting others in reaching their own health goals. From renowned wellness experts as visiting teachers to the convenience of their online learning platform, this school has changed my life, and I believe it will do the same for you. I invite you to learn more about the Institute for Integrative Nutrition and explore how the Health Coach Training Program can help you transform your life. Feel free to contact me to hear more about my personal experience in Blossom's FearLess Facebook Group or @BlossomsFearLess. Or call (844) 315.8546 to learn more.

Blossom's FearLess journal in an integrative health coach In a book. This therapeutic journal is designed to guide you toward your transformation. It is a book that only you can write, designed to help you discover what your life was meant to be.

Transformation comes from within. Join me on this path toward the discovery of your Higher Self. It has always been there, but at times, it may seem to be dormant or restoring itself. With this commitment to self-exploration, you are choosing transformation, to live in grace-filled flow.

Tamara Hall Fuchs is a former neurodiversity specialist who has created this therapeutic journal to support you in becoming your best Self.

 Blossom's FearLess

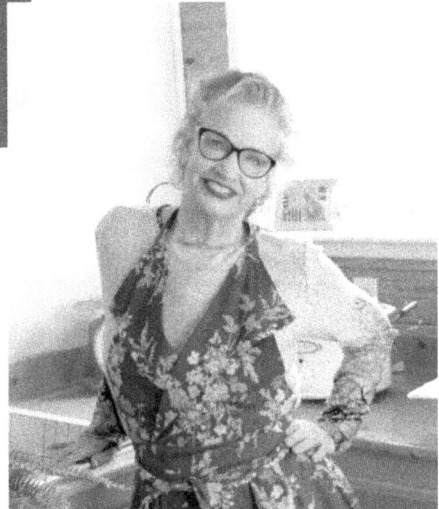

 @BlossomsFearLess

This journal will help youFind your purpose, define who you are, what you want, and how to get there. This journal will do the following;
- Provide tools to help you let go of what no longer serves you and discover new tools that do;
- Lead a guided journey to your authentic Self, untamed and glorious;
- Discover your inner strength to tackle the hard stuff;
- Introduce and support vital life skills, such as problem-solving, decision-making, managing interpersonal relationships, health and wellness tracking, and so much more!

www.ingramcontent.com/pod-product-compliance
Lightning Source LLC
Chambersburg PA
CBHW080547270326
41929CB00019B/3221